D1380306

Do You Have Anxiety? Check Your Symptoms

Anxiety appears in different forms for different people. You may find that anxiety affects your thoughts, behaviours, and feelings. Some of the more common symptoms are listed as follows:

You're _thinking_ anxiously if you're . . .

- Making dire predictions about the future
- Thinking you can't cope
- Frequently worrying about pleasing people
- Thinking that you need to be perfect
- Having excessive concerns about not being in control
- Having difficulty concentrating

You're _behaving_ anxiously if you're . . .

- Avoiding many social events
- Leaving situations that make you anxious
- Never taking reasonable risks
- Staying away from feared objects or events, such as flying or spiders

You're _feeling_ anxious if you have . . .

- Butterflies in your stomach
- Dizziness
- Muscle tension
- A racing heart
- A shaky feeling
- Sweaty palms

Warning: The physical symptoms of anxiety may result from medical problems. If you have a number of these symptoms, please see a doctor for a checkup.

Three Quick Ways to Reduce Anxiety

- Engaging in 20 minutes of aerobic exercise
- Taking a walk with or without a friend
- Soaking in a warm bath

See Chapter 10 for more suggestions on reducing anxiety.

Dealing with Your Anxious Thoughts

When your mind fills with worries and concerns, try asking yourself these questions:

- How will I look at this concern six months from now?
- Have I had this worry before only to discover that what I worried about never actually occurred?
- What evidence exists to either support or contradict my worry?
- If a friend of mine had this thought, what advice would I give?
- If the worst happens, could I find a way to cope with it?

See Chapter 5 for more questions.

Overcoming Anxiety
For Dummies®

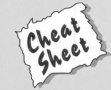

Cheat Sheet

Conquering Your Anxious Behaviour

When you find that you're avoiding important life events or opportunities, it's time to take action. Try these suggestions:

1. **Analyse what you're avoiding.**

   What is it about the situation that frightens you? If you don't know, think through what would happen if you stayed there, when you desperately felt you just had to leave.

2. **Break your avoidance into little steps.**

   For example, social gatherings come in all sizes and degrees of difficulty, from small family affairs up to large corporate events.

3. **Rank those small steps from least to most distressing.**

   You may not feel anxious about family gatherings, but the work's Christmas party makes you more anxious, and a party full of people that you don't know well – your partner's work do – terrifies you.

4. **Take small steps and conquer each step before moving on.**

   See Chapter 8 for details on coming to terms with your fears.

Calming Your Anxious Feelings

When you feel anxious all over, with sensations like sweaty hands, a shaky voice, a racing heart, or an upset stomach, try a few relaxing breaths:

1. **Put your hand on your abdomen.**
2. **Take a slow, deep breath and notice your abdomen expanding.**
3. **Hold that breath for five or six seconds.**
4. **Slowly breathe out and let your shoulders droop.**
5. **As you exhale, say the word 'relax' to yourself.**
6. **Repeat this type of breath ten times.**

   See Chapter 12 for more relaxation techniques.

For Dummies: Bestselling Book Series for Beginners

About the Authors

Elaine Iljon Foreman, MSc, AFBPSs, is a consultant chartered clinical psychologist and a member of the British Psychological Society, the British Association for Behavioural and Cognitive Psychotherapy, and the British Travel Health Association. Elaine specialises in the treatment of fear of flying, as well as other anxiety-related problems, including panic attacks, claustrophobia, agoraphobia, and specific phobias. She applies cognitive behavioural therapy techniques to assist people in overcoming a wide range of anxieties, even when they have had long histories of these problems. Elaine has developed highly specialised treatment programmes for a wide variety of anxiety disorders based on over 25 years of clinical experience and on her continuing research and development of cognitive behaviour therapy.

Invitations to present her findings have taken Elaine to Europe, the Americas, Australia, and the Far East. She co-ordinates international research into fear of flying, and has her own specialist consultancy practice. Her Web site is at www.freedomtofly.biz.

Charles H Elliott, PhD, is a clinical psychologist and a member of the faculty at the Fielding Graduate Institute. He is a Founding Fellow in the Academy of Cognitive Therapy, an internationally recognized organisation that certifies cognitive therapists for treating anxiety, panic attacks, and other emotional disorders. In his private clinical practice, he specialises in the treatment of anxiety and mood disorders. Elliott is the former president of the New Mexico Society of Biofeedback and Behavioral Medicine. He previously served as Director of Mental Health Consultation-Liaison Service at the University of Oklahoma Health Sciences Center. He later was an Associate Professor in the psychiatry department at the University of New Mexico School of Medicine. In addition, he has written many articles and book chapters in the area of cognitive behavior therapies. He has made numerous presentations nationally and internationally on new developments in assessment and therapy of emotional disorders. He is co-author of *Why Can't I Get What I Want?* (Davies-Black, 1998; A Behavioral Science Book Club Selection), *Why Can't I Be the Parent I Want to Be?* (New Harbinger Publications, 1999), and *Hollow Kids: Recapturing the Soul of a Generation Lost to the Self-Esteem Myth* (Prima, 2001).

Laura L Smith, PhD, is a clinical psychologist at Presbyterian Behavioral Medicine, Albuquerque, New Mexico. At Presbyterian, she specialises in the assessment and treatment of both adults and children with anxiety and other mood disorders. She is an adjunct faculty member at the Fielding Graduate Institute. Formerly, she was the clinical supervisor for a regional educational cooperative. In addition, she has presented on new developments in cognitive therapy to both national and international audiences. Dr Smith is co-author of *Hollow Kids* (Prima, 2001) and *Why Can't I Be the Parent I Want to Be?* (New Harbinger Publications, 1999).

Dedication

From Elaine: This book is dedicated to Helga and Nickie Iljon, with special thanks to Sharon Malyan, a real source of inspiration to her students, friends, and most of all, family.

From Charles and Laura: We dedicate this book to our children: Alli, Brian, Sara, and Trevor. And to our parents: William Thomas Smith (1914-1999), Edna Louise Smith, Joe Bond Elliott, and Suzanne Wieder Elliott.

Authors' Acknowledgements

Elaine would like to offer special thanks to Dr Daniel McQueen, BMedSci MBBS MRCP MRCPsych, Specialist Registrar in Psychotherapy at the Cassel Hospital and West Middlesex University Hospital, for his invaluable help with Chapter 15. In addition, Freda Miller, BSc (Exon), BSc (Wales) MNIMH, MCPP, offered valuable input into Chapter 14, which is much appreciated. Thanks also to Alison Yates and Simon Bell at John Wiley & Sons, Ltd.

Charles and Laura would like to thank, as usual, our families and friends, once again neglected.

Thanks also to our enthusiastic agents, Ed and Elizabeth Knappman, who have shown consistent faith in our writing. We appreciate the expertise and professionalism of our editors at John Wiley & Sons, Inc.; special thanks to Norm Crampton, Esmeralda St. Clair, and Natasha Graf.

Thanks to Audrey Hite for keeping the house in order, Scott Love for designing our Web site and keeping our computers up and running, Diana Montoya-Boyer for keeping us organised and gathering materials, and Karen Villanueva, our personal publicist.

Finally, we appreciate all that we've learned from our many clients over the years. They have provided us with a greater understanding of the problems those with anxiety face, as well as the brave struggle involved in overcoming anxiety.

Publisher's Acknowledgements

We're proud of this book; please send us your comments through our Dummies online registration form located at www.dummies.com/register/.

Some of the people who helped bring this book to market include the following:

Acquisitions, Editorial, and Media Development

Project Editor: Simon Bell

Commissioning Editor: Alison Yates

Content Editor: Steve Edwards

Copy Editor: Charlie Wilson

Technical Editor: Dr Cosmo Hallstrom, MB,ChB, DPM, MRCPsych, MD, MRCP, FRCPsych

Executive Editor: Jason Dunne

Executive Project Editor: Martin Tribe

Cover Photo: Joson/zefa/Corbis

Cartoons: Ed McLachlan

Composition Services

Project Coordinator: Jennifer Theriot

Layout and Graphics: Carl Byers, Alicia B. South, Christine Williams, Erin Zeltner

Proofreader: Laura Albert

Indexer: Aptara

Anniversary Logo Design: Richard J. Pacifico

Publishing and Editorial for Consumer Dummies

>   **Diane Graves Steele,** Vice President and Publisher, Consumer Dummies

>   **Joyce Pepple,** Acquisitions Director, Consumer Dummies

>   **Kristin A. Cocks,** Product Development Director, Consumer Dummies

>   **Michael Spring,** Vice President and Publisher, Travel

>   **Kelly Regan,** Editorial Director, Travel

Publishing for Technology Dummies

>   **Andy Cummings,** Vice President and Publisher, Dummies Technology/General User

Composition Services

>   **Gerry Fahey,** Vice President of Production Services

>   **Debbie Stailey,** Director of Composition Services

Contents at a Glance

Table of Contents

Introduction

· ·

Growing up today, children and parents face yet more worries and anxieties added to the old. Children have always been taught, 'Don't talk to strangers', and there are new messages such as 'Report suspicious packages'. High profile terrorist incidents give a heightened sense of danger and vulnerability. To some extent we all worry, and there are sometimes good reasons to.

But although today's world gives people plenty to worry about, so it always has. Just as we don't want to become victims of terrorism, for example, we can't let ourselves become victims of anxiety. Anxiety clouds thinking and weakens people's resolve to live life to the fullest. Some anxiety is realistic and inescapable; yet people can keep it from dominating their lives. Even under duress, everyone can preserve a degree of serenity, and hold on to their humanity, common sense, strength, and zest for life. We can all still love and laugh.

Because we, the authors, believe in our collective resilience, we take a humorous and at times irreverent approach to conquering anxiety. Our message is based on sound, scientifically proven methods. But we won't bore you with the scientific details. Instead, we present a clear, rapid-fire set of strategies for beating back anxiety and winning the war against worry.

About This Book

We have three goals in writing this book. First, we want you to understand just what anxiety is and its different forms. Second, we think that knowing what's good about anxiety and what's bad about it is good for you. Finally, we cover what you're probably most interested in – discovering how to overcome your anxiety or how to help someone else who has anxiety.

Unlike most books, you don't have to start on page one and read straight through. Use the extensive Table of Contents to pick and choose what you want to read. Don't worry about reading parts in any particular order. For example, if you really don't want much information about the who, what, when, where, and why's of anxiety, and whether you have it, go ahead and skip Part I. However, we encourage you to at least skim Part I because it contains fascinating facts and information as well as ideas for getting started.

What Not to Read

Not only do you not have to read each and every chapter in order or at all, you don't have to look at each and every icon or aside. We try to give you plenty of current information and facts about anxiety. Some may not interest you, so don't get too anxious about skipping around.

Foolish Assumptions

Who may pick up this book? We assume, probably not too foolishly, that you or someone you love suffers from some type of problem with anxiety. We also believe that you want information to help tame tension and conquer anxiety. Finally, we imagine that you're curious about a variety of helpful strategies to choose from that can fit your lifestyle and personality.

How This Book Is Organised

Overcoming Anxiety For Dummies is organised into six parts and 22 chapters. Here, we tell you a little about each part.

Part I: Detecting and Exposing Anxiety

In these first two chapters, you find out a great deal about anxiety, ranging from who gets it to why people become anxious. We explain the different kinds of anxiety disorders, and we tell you who is most susceptible and why.

In Chapter 3, we help you to overcome the obstacles to change. You discover the most common reasons that people resist working on their anxiety, and what to do about it if you find yourself stuck. Chapter 4 gives you ways to keep track of your progress.

Part II: Understanding Thought Remedies

In Part II, you see how thinking contributes to anxious feelings. We show you a variety of proven strategies that can transform anxious thoughts into calm thoughts. And you discover how the words that you use can increase anxiety and how simply changing your vocabulary decreases anxiety.

Part III: Acting Against Anxiety

One of the best ways to tackle anxiety is by taking action. No place for cowards here. We show you how to look your fears full in the face and conquer them. We also explore other anti-anxiety actions, such as changing your lifestyle.

Part IV: Focusing on Feeling

In this part, we offer a treasure trove of ideas for quelling anxious feelings. These ideas range from special breathing techniques to imaginary journeys – using various means to relax your body and mind. We give you the latest research findings on what works and what doesn't among herbs, supplements, and medication.

Part V: Helping Others with Anxiety

What do you do when someone you love worries too much? We give you the tools to understand the differences between normal fear and anxiety in children. We also provide some simple guidelines to help anxious youngsters. Next, we look at how you can help an adult close to you who suffers from anxiety. As a coach or simply by providing encouragement, you can help your friend or family member conquer anxiety.

Part VI: The Part of Tens

If you're looking for a quick fix or just to review, take a look at these helpful lists. You can read about Ten Ways to Stop Anxiety Quickly, Ten Typical Tactics Doomed to Fail, Ten Ways to Deal with Relapse, and Ten Signs That You Need Professional Help.

Icons Used in This Book

This icon represents a particular tip for getting rid of anxiety.

The Anxiety Quiz icon lets you know when it's time to take a quiz. (Don't worry; the quizzes aren't scored, but they do help you organise your thinking about anxiety.)

This icon appears when we want your attention. Please read for essential information.

 The Tip icon alerts you to important insights or clarifications.

 These icons appear when you need to be careful or seek professional help.

Where to Go from Here

Overcoming Anxiety For Dummies offers you the best advice based on scientific research in the area of anxiety disorders. We know that if you practise the techniques and strategies provided throughout this book, you're pretty likely to feel calmer. For most people, this book should be a complete guide to fighting fear and enabling you to progress from stress to strength.

However, some stubborn forms of anxiety need more detailed, professional attention. If your anxiety and worry significantly get in the way of your work or play, you need to get help. Start with your family doctor. Anxiety can be conquered: Don't give up.

Part I
Detecting and Exposing Anxiety

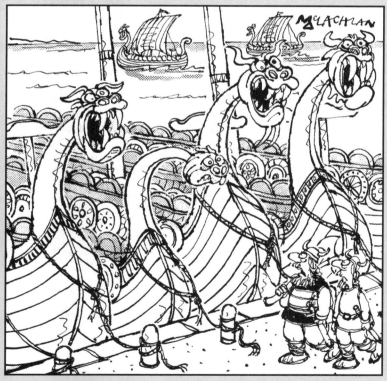

'. . . that's Ragnar the Bloodaxe's, that's Sven the
Bonecrusher's, and this one's Eric the Anxious's . . .'

In this part . . .

*E*xploring the ins and outs of anxiety, we discuss the anxiety epidemic and show how anxiety affects the entire body. In this part, you can find all the major categories of anxiety disorders, and get an overview of some things you can do to reduce anxiety. You'll discover how you can easily get stuck tackling your anxiety, and we tell you how to prevent this from happening. Finally, we give you ways to chart your anxiety, so you can look forward to the progress that you'll surely make towards reducing it.

Chapter 1

Analysing and Attacking Anxiety

Anxiety, stress, and worries. Everyone has these experiences. They are part of normal life – no way can we expect to go through life without experiencing them. But sometimes they get out of hand. Then anxiety causes pain, for a surprising number of people. Anxiety can create havoc in the home, destroy relationships, make employees lose time from work, and prevent people from living full, productive lives.

When people talk about their anxiety, you may hear any one or all of the following descriptions:

✔ I just can't find the right words to describe my feelings. It's like dread and doom, but a thousand times worse. I want to scream, cry for help, but I'm paralysed. It's the worst feeling in the world.

✔ When my panic attacks begin, I feel tightness in my chest. It's as though I'm drowning or suffocating, and I begin to sweat; the fear is overwhelming. I feel like I'm going to die, and I have to sit down because I'm convinced I'm going to faint.

✔ I'm lonely. I've always been painfully shy. I want friends, but I'm too embarrassed to contact anyone. I guess I feel anyone I call will think that I'm not worth talking to.

✔ I wake up worried every day, even on the weekends. I never feel I've caught up – there's always a list and always responsibility. I worry all the time. Sometimes, when it's really bad, I think about going to sleep and never waking up.

In this chapter, we talk about symptoms of anxiety. We clarify the costs of anxiety – both to you personally and to society. We briefly overview the treatments presented in greater detail in later chapters and give you a tool for choosing the one that may fit your personality best as a way to begin overcoming anxiety. You also get a glimpse of how you can help if someone you care about suffers with anxiety.

Anxiety: You Can't Escape It

Anxiety is the most common of all the so-called mental disorders. Estimates suggest that around 6.5 million people in the UK suffer from an anxiety disorder in any given year, and some calculate that as many as 25 per cent may suffer from an anxiety disorder at one point or another over a lifetime. Statistics around the world vary somewhat from country to country, but anxiety is the most common mental disorder worldwide. And even if you don't have an actual anxiety disorder, you may experience more anxiety than you want. In other words, you definitely aren't alone if you have unwanted anxiety.

And the number of people troubled by anxiety has grown over the years. Why?

Life has never been as complicated as it is today. The working week keeps getting longer rather than shorter, despite legislation. Divorce, separation, and combining families create increased stresses for you to manage. Television news blasts the latest horrors into your living room. Newspapers and magazines chronicle crime, war, and corruption. Terrorism has landed on our shores and escalated to new heights. The media's portrayal of these modern plagues includes full-colour images with unprecedented, graphic detail.

Unfortunately, as stressful and anxiety-arousing as the world is today, only a minority of those suffering from anxiety seek treatment. That's a problem because anxiety causes not only emotional pain and distress, but even death, given that anxiety sometimes contributes to suicide. Furthermore, anxiety costs society as a whole billions of pounds.

Calculating the Costs of Anxiety

Anxiety costs. It costs the sufferer in emotional, physical, and financial terms. But anxiety doesn't stop there. Anxiety also incurs a financial burden for everyone. Stress, worry, and anxiety disrupt relationships, work, leisure, and family.

What does anxiety cost you?

Obviously, if you have a problem with anxiety, you experience the cost of distressed, anxious feelings. Anxiety feels dreadful. You don't need to read a book to know that. But did you know that untreated anxiety takes its toll in other ways as well? These costs include

- **A physical toll:** Higher blood pressure, tension headaches, and gastrointestinal symptoms can affect your body. In fact, recent research found that certain types of chronic anxiety disorders change the makeup of your brain's structures. Links have also been found between anxiety, stress, and heart disease.

- **A toll on your kids:** Parents with anxiety more often have anxious children. This is due in part to genetics, but it's also because children learn from observation.

- **Gaining weight:** Anxiety and stress increase the stress hormone *cortisol*. Cortisol causes fat storage in the abdominal area, thus increasing the risk of heart disease and stroke. Stress also leads to increased eating.

- **More doctors' appointments:** Those with anxiety frequently experience worrisome physical symptoms. In addition, anxious people often worry a great deal about their health.

- **Relationship problems:** People with anxiety frequently feel irritable. Sometimes, they withdraw emotionally or do the opposite and dependently cling to their partners.

- **Sick leave:** Those with anxiety disorders miss work more often than other people.

Adding up the cost to society

Anxiety costs many billions of pounds worldwide. While the costs of mental health problems for UK society are estimated at £77 billion annually, in the US, the Government reports that anxiety costs more than depression, schizophrenia, or any other emotional problem. In the UK, 50 per cent of all working days lost through mental illness are because of anxiety and stress. Even countries that spend little on mental health care incur substantial costs from anxiety disorders. These costs include

- Decreased productivity
- Healthcare costs, including medication
- Self-medication in the form of drugs and alcohol

Decreased productivity can be due to the adverse effects of anxiety on a person's health, or even to suicide. But the financial loss from sick leave and healthcare costs doesn't include the money lost to substance abuse. Many of those with anxiety disorders use alcohol and drugs in order to deal with their anxiety, only to then experience the additional problems of substance abuse. Thus, directly and indirectly, anxiety has a colossal toll on both the person who experiences it as well as society at large.

Recognising the Symptoms of Anxiety

You may be unaware that you suffer from anxiety or an anxiety disorder. That's because anxiety involves a rather wide range of symptoms. Each person experiences slightly different symptoms. And your own specific symptoms determine what kind of anxiety disorder you may have. We discuss the various types of anxiety disorders in detail in Chapter 2.

For now, you should know that some signs of anxiety appear in the form of *thoughts* or *beliefs*. Other indications of anxiety manifest themselves in *bodily sensations*. Still other symptoms show up in various kinds of anxious *behaviours*. Some people experience anxiety signs in all three ways, while others only notice their anxiety in one or two areas.

Thinking anxiously

In Part II, we discuss anxious thinking in great detail. For starters, people with anxiety generally think differently from other people. Look out for the following: You're probably thinking anxiously if you experience

- ✔ **Approval addiction:** If you're an approval addict, you worry a great deal about what other people think about you.

- ✔ **Living in the future and predicting the worst:** When you do this, you think about everything that lies ahead and assume the worst possible outcome, a type of thinking known as *catastrophising*.

- ✔ **Magnification:** People who magnify the importance of negative events usually feel more anxious than other people do.

- ✔ **Perfectionism:** If you're a perfectionist, you assume that any mistake means total failure.

- ✔ **Poor concentration:** Anxious people routinely report that they struggle to focus their thoughts. Short-term memory sometimes suffers as well.

- ✔ **Racing thoughts:** When thoughts race, they run through your mind in a stream of almost uncontrollable worry and concern.

Finding anxiety in your body

Almost all people with severe anxiety experience a range of physical effects. These sensations don't simply occur in your head; they're as real as this book you're holding. The responses to anxiety vary considerably from person to person and include

- ✔ Accelerated heart beat
- ✔ A spike in blood pressure
- ✔ Blurred vision
- ✔ Dizziness
- ✔ Fatigue
- ✔ Feelings of unreality
- ✔ Gastrointestinal upset
- ✔ General aches and pains
- ✔ Muscle tension or spasms
- ✔ Sweating

These are simply the temporary effects that anxiety exerts on your body. Chronic anxiety left untreated can pose serious risks to your health. We discuss the general health effects in greater detail in Chapter 2.

Behaving anxiously

We have three words to describe anxious behaviour: avoidance, avoidance, and avoidance. Anxious people inevitably attempt to get away, and stay away, from the things that make them anxious. Whether it's snakes, heights, crowds, motorways, parties, paying bills, reminders of bad times, or public speaking, anxious people search for escape routes.

One of the most common and obvious examples of anxiety-induced avoidance is how people react to their phobias. Have you ever seen the response of a spider-phobic when confronting one of the beasties? Usually, the phobic beats a hasty retreat.

In the short run, avoidance decreases anxiety. It can make you feel a little better. However, in the long run, avoidance actually maintains and heightens anxiety. We discuss the role that avoidance plays in increasing your anxiety in Chapter 2, and we give you ways of confronting avoidance in Chapter 8.

Seeking Help for Your Anxiety

As we said earlier in this chapter, most people choose to simply live with anxiety rather than seek help. Some people worry that treatment won't work. Or they believe that the medication is the only effective treatment they have, and they hate the possibility of side effects, as well as feeling they should be able to manage on their own and not be so weak as to need help. While certain people are concerned that others might think less of them or mock them if they seek help and are terrified of the embarrassment, others worry about the availability and costs of treatment – the NHS usually has long waiting lists, and private therapy can be expensive.

Well, stop adding worry to worry. You can significantly reduce your anxiety through a variety of interesting strategies. Many of these don't have to cost a single penny. And if one doesn't work, try another. Most people find that at least a couple of the approaches that we review in this book work for them.

Untreated anxiety may cause long-term health problems. So not doing something about your anxiety doesn't make sense.

Matching symptoms and therapies

Anxiety symptoms appear in three different spheres:

- **Thinking symptoms:** The thoughts that run through your mind.
- **Behaving symptoms:** The things you do in response to anxiety.
- **Feeling symptoms:** How your body reacts to anxiety.

You may well experience symptoms from all these groups but find one more powerful and disturbing than the others.

The following sections address treatment for these three kinds of symptom.

Thinking therapies

One of the most effective treatments for a wide range of emotional problems, known as *cognitive therapy,* deals with the way you think about, perceive, and interpret everything that's important to you including

- Your views about yourself
- The events that happen to you in life
- Your future

When people feel unusually anxious and worried, they almost inevitably distort the way they think about things, especially those things that are important to them. That distortion actually causes much of their anxiety.

For example, **Susan** is in her first year of university. She gets physically ill before every exam. She throws up, has diarrhoea, and her heart races. She fantasises that she will fail each and every exam she takes and eventually she will be thrown out. Yet, her lowest essay mark to date has been a B–. A cognitive approach would help her capture the negative predictions and catastrophic outcomes that run through her mind. This approach would guide her to search for evidence about her true performance and gain a more realistic view of her chances of actually failing.

As simple as this approach sounds, hundreds of studies have found that it works well to reduce anxiety. The approach is tailored to the specific difficulties that a person has. Using the principles of cognitive therapy, individualised strategies are developed to enable the person to overcome her problem. Part II of this book describes various cognitive or thinking therapy techniques.

Behaving therapies

Another highly effective type of therapy is known as *behaviour therapy*. As the name suggests, this approach deals with actions you can take and behaviours you can incorporate to alleviate your anxiety. Some actions are fairly straightforward:

- Simplify your life (see Chapter 9)
- Get more exercise (see Chapter 10)
- Get more sleep (see Chapter 11)

On the other hand, one type of behaviour therapy that is likely to be very effective, but which can feel a little scary, is *graded exposure* – breaking your fears down into small steps and facing them one at a time. Exposure, however, is a bit more complicated and does involve a little more than this statement indicates, so turn to Chapter 8 for more about exposure.

Feeling therapies

Anxiety sets off a whirlwind of distressing physical symptoms, such as a racing heartbeat, upset stomach, muscle tension, sweating, dizziness, and so on. We have a variety of suggestions for helping to quell these symptoms.

You may prefer herbal remedies. If you want more information about herbs for anxiety, see Chapter 14. Some of these herbs appear to work pretty well, while others are more hype than hope.

If you have five minutes to spare in your daily schedule, you can try a number of our five-minute strategies for relaxation. The key to all relaxation techniques is simple – if you're relaxed, it's much harder to feel anxious. See Chapter 12 for quick and easy ways to relax.

On the other hand, some people choose to take medication for anxiety. If that's your choice, Chapter 15 tells you about the available options. The decision to take medication involves a variety of costs and benefits that you should weigh up carefully. We give you the tools for making this decision.

In the following anxiety quiz, tick all the items that apply to you. If you tick an equal number of items for two or more categories, ask yourself which one seems most like you and start from there. Developments in therapy have meant that now a number of techniques from different areas are combined to be even more effective. *Cognitive behavioural therapy*, or CBT, is the best known of these newer developments. It takes into account thought, behaviour, and feelings. For more detail on what CBT can do for you, check out Chapter 5. You should also grab a copy of *Cognitive Behavioural Therapy For Dummies*, by Rob Willson and Rhena Branch (Wiley).

Thinkers

For more on being a thinker, see Part II (Chapters 5–7).

- ✔ I like to analyse problems.
- ✔ I like to carefully weigh up the pros and cons.
- ✔ I enjoy dealing with facts.
- ✔ I like to be logical.
- ✔ I like to plan things in advance.

Doers

If this quiz reveals you to be a doer, turn to Part III (Chapters 8–11) for more about doers.

- ✔ If I have a problem, I take action right away.
- ✔ I love getting things done.
- ✔ I'm energetic.
- ✔ I'm an active person.
- ✔ I hate sitting still with nothing to do.

Feelers

If you're a feeler, be sure to read Part IV (Chapters 12–16).

> ✔ I am always aware of every discomfort in my body.
>
> ✔ I hate the feeling of anxiety.
>
> ✔ I love to immerse myself in the arts.
>
> ✔ Music speaks to me.
>
> ✔ I love the feeling of a massage or a hot bath.

Finding the right help

Because you're interested in this book, we imagine either you or someone you know suffers from anxiety. And you'd probably like to tackle anxiety on your own. This *is* a self-help book after all.

Self-help does work. In fact, a number of studies support the idea that people can deal with important, difficult problems without seeking the services of a professional. People clearly benefit from self-help. They get better and they stay better. In fact, a new scheme has been rolled out to more than 45 UK Health Authorities which enables doctors to prescribe specific self-help books. You simply take the prescription to your local library, and the librarian fills it with the self-help book prescribed. Computer-based self-help programmes can also be effective and are increasingly being offered through doctors' surgeries and over the Internet. If you find your own via the Internet, do check with your doctor that it is one of the ones that has been tested and found useful. (See 'Resources' in the Appendix.)

Sometimes, however, self-help efforts fall short. In Chapter 22 we provide you with ten critical signs that indicate a likely need for professional help. If you do need a professional consultation, many qualified therapists will work with you on the ideas conveyed in this book.

Most mental health professionals appreciate the comprehensive nature of the material in this book, and the fact that the majority of the strategies are based on well-proven methods. If research has yet to support the value of a particular approach, we take care to let you know that. At the same time, in Chapter 20, we review ten over-hyped techniques of dubious value. That's because we think that you're much better off sticking with strategies known to work and avoiding those that don't.

Friends and family represent one more source of possible help. In Chapters 17 and 18, we discuss how to help a child or an adult who has anxiety. If you're asking a friend or family member to help, you may both want to read that section, and possibly more. Sometimes, friends and family can help you even if you're also working with a professional and making your own efforts.

Whichever sources, techniques, and/or strategies you select, overcoming anxiety is one of the most rewarding challenges that you ever undertake. The endeavour may scare you at first, and the going may start slow and have its ups and downs, but stick with it, and we're confident that you'll find a way out of the quicksand of anxiety onto the solid ground of serenity.

Chapter 2

Examining Anxiety: What's Normal, What's Not

The physical symptoms of anxiety can be a part of normal, everyday experience. But sometimes they signal something more serious. Think about yourself. Have you ever thought that you were suffering a nervous breakdown or worried that you were going crazy? Perhaps you felt you were having a heart attack?

In this chapter, we help you work out what's going on – whether you're suffering from an anxiety disorder, normal anxiety, or something else. You'll also see how your body responds to anxiety.

To demonstrate the difference between an actual anxiety disorder and a normal reaction, read the following description and imagine ten minutes in the life of Sandy.

At first, **Sandy** feels restless and slightly bored. Standing, she shifts her weight from foot to foot. Walking forward a little, she notices a slight tightening of her chest. Her breathing quickens. She feels an odd mixture of excitement and mounting tension. She sits down and does her best to relax, but the anxiety continues to intensify. Her body suddenly jerks forward; she grips the sides of her seat and clenches her teeth to choke back a scream. Her stomach feels like it's rising up into her throat. Then it settles down. She feels her heart race and her face flush. Once more her stomach seems to rise up into her throat. Sandy's emotions run wild. Dizziness, fear, and a rushing sensation overtake her. It all comes in waves, one after the other.

Name that phobia!

Phobias are one of the most common types of anxiety disorders, and we discuss them in detail in Chapter 2. A phobia is an excessive, disproportionate fear of a relatively harmless situation or thing. Sometimes the phobia poses some risk, but the person's reaction clearly exceeds the danger. Do you know the technical names for phobias? Draw arrows from the common name of each phobia to the corresponding technical name. See how many you get right. The answers are printed upside down at the bottom of this exercise.

Be careful if you have *triskaidekaphobia* (fear of the number 13) because we're giving you thirteen phobias to match!

Technical name	Means a fear of _____
1. Ophidiophobia	A. Growing old
2. Zoophobia	B. Sleep
3. Gerascophobia	C. The mind
4. Acrophobia	D. Imperfection
5. Lachanophobia	E. Snakes
6. Hypnophobia	F. Fear
7. Atelophobia	G. New things
8. Phobophobia	H. Animals
9. Sesquipedalophobia	I. Small things
10. Neophobia	J. Mirrors
11. Psychophobia	K. Heights
12. Tapinophobia	L. Long words
13. Eisoptrophobia	M. Vegetables

Answers: 1-e, 2-h, 3-a, 4-k, 5-m, 6-b, 7-d, 8-f, 9-l, 10-g, 11-c, 12-i, 13-j.

You may wonder what's wrong with poor Sandy. Perhaps she has an anxiety disorder. Or could she be having a nervous breakdown – and maybe even be going crazy?

But Sandy's just spent those last ten minutes, plus many more, at an amusement park. First, she queued to buy a ticket and felt bored. Then she handed her ticket to the attendant and strapped herself into a roller coaster. After that, well, no doubt you now understand the rest of her experience. Sandy has no anxiety disorder, she isn't suffering a nervous breakdown, and she isn't going mad. As her story illustrates, the symptoms of anxiety can be a normal reaction to life events.

Presenting the Seven Main Types of Anxiety

Anxiety comes in various forms. The word *anxious* is derived from the Latin word *angere,* meaning to press tightly, strangle, or choke. A sense of choking or tightening in the throat or chest is a common symptom of anxiety. However, anxiety also involves other symptoms, such as sweating, trembling, nausea, and a racing heartbeat. Anxiety may also involve fears – fear of losing control and fear of illness or of dying. In addition, people with excessive anxiety avoid various situations, people, animals, or objects to an unnecessary degree. Psychologists and psychiatrists have compiled a list of seven major categories of anxiety disorders as follows:

- ✔ Generalised anxiety disorder (GAD)
- ✔ Social phobia
- ✔ Panic disorder
- ✔ Agoraphobia
- ✔ Specific phobia
- ✔ Post-traumatic stress disorder (PTSD)
- ✔ Obsessive-compulsive disorder (OCD)

In this chapter, we describe the signs and indications of each of the major types of anxiety disorders. Medical students are renowned for thinking that they have developed every new disease they study. Readers of psychology books sometimes do the same thing. Don't panic if you or someone you love experiences some of these symptoms. Almost everyone has a few of them.

You don't need a full-blown diagnosis to feel that you have some trouble with anxiety. Many people have more anxiety than they want but don't completely meet the criteria of having a diagnosable anxiety disorder.

Only a mental health professional can tell you for certain what type of anxiety you have, because various other disorders can look similar, including medical problems discussed later in this chapter in the section 'Investigating medical conditions with accompanying anxiety'.

Although we provide the major signs and symptoms of each type of anxiety so that you can get a general idea of which category your anxiety may fall into, to really understand where your particular anxiety fits, you need to see a professional (see Chapter 22). If you do seek professional help, the ideas in this book can still assist you in alleviating your problems with anxiety.

Generalised anxiety disorder: The common cold of anxiety

Some people refer to *generalised anxiety disorder* as the common cold of anxiety disorders. Generalised anxiety disorder, also known as GAD, afflicts more people throughout the world than any other anxiety disorder. So if you or a loved one has it, you're in good company. GAD involves a long-lasting, almost constant state of tension and worry. Realistic worries don't mean you have GAD. For example, if you worry about money and you've just lost your job, that's not GAD – it's a real-life problem. But if you constantly worry about money and your name is Bill Gates, you just may have GAD!

You may have GAD if you've experienced anxiety almost daily for the last six months. You try to stop worrying but you just can't. *And* you frequently experience a number of the following problems:

- ✔ You feel restless; often irritable, on edge, fidgety, or keyed up.
- ✔ You get tired easily.
- ✔ Your muscles feel tense, especially in your back, neck, or shoulders.
- ✔ You have difficulty concentrating, falling asleep, or staying asleep.

Not everyone experiences anxiety in exactly the same way. That's why only a professional can actually make a diagnosis. Some people complain about other problems, such as twitching, trembling, shortness of breath, sweating, dry mouth, stomach upset, feeling shaky, being easily startled, and having difficulty swallowing. They fail to realise that they actually suffer from GAD.

The following profile offers an example of what GAD is all about.

On the Underground train, **Brian** taps his foot nervously. He arches his back to stretch his tight shoulder muscles and checks his watch, worrying that he may be three or four minutes late for work. He hates coming in late. He didn't sleep much last night because thoughts about the presentation of his latest project repeatedly invaded his sleep. One preoccupation or another usually disturbs Brian's sleep. Struggling to concentrate on the newspaper that he's holding, he realises that he can't remember what he's just read.

When Brian gets to work, he snaps at his new assistant. After he loses his temper with her, he feels immediate remorse and angrily tells himself off, increasing his anxiety further. His colleagues often tell him to keep cool. His performance has always exceeded his employer's expectations, so he objectively has no reason to worry about his job. Nevertheless, worry he does. Brian suffers from GAD.

The paradox of social phobia

Because of the expectation and fear of experiencing humiliation, those with social phobia withdraw and avoid social situations whenever possible. When forced into such encounters, they inhibit their actions in order to avoid saying or doing something that they believe will be seen as stupid. They often avoid eye contact, stand alone, contribute little to conversations, and generally look stiff and ill at ease.

Unfortunately, this fear of expressing themselves sometimes makes social phobics appear unfriendly, cold, distant, and/or self-centred. Social phobics actually experience intense fear in these circumstances and react with surprise to feedback that they seem self-centred and unfriendly. Sometimes, if they do realise that others perceive them as unfriendly, this only fuels the phobia and convinces them that people won't and don't like them, and that they don't know how to interact successfully. In other words, a vicious cycle is created – the more social phobics try to avoid negative reactions, the more negatively others react.

Social phobia – avoiding people

Those with *social phobia* fear exposure to public scrutiny. They frequently dread interviews, performing, speaking in groups or even one to one, going to parties, meeting new people, entering groups, using the telephone, writing a cheque in front of others, eating in public, and/or interacting with those in authority. They see these situations as painful, because they expect to receive humiliating or shameful judgements from others. Social phobics often believe that they're somehow defective and inadequate; thus, they assume that they'll mess things up, for instance muff their lines, spill their drinks, shake hands with clammy palms, or commit any of a number of social *faux pas* and thus embarrass themselves.

 We all feel uncomfortable or nervous from time to time, especially in new situations. So if you've been experiencing social fears for less than six months, you may well not have social phobia. A short-term fear of socialising may be a temporary reaction to a new stress – moving to a new area or starting a new job. However, you may have social phobia if you experience the following symptoms for a prolonged period of time:

- You fear being in situations with unfamiliar people or where you may be observed or evaluated in some way.

- When forced into an uncomfortable social situation, your physical symptoms and scary thoughts can feel overwhelming. For example, if you fear public speaking, your voice shakes, and your knees tremble the moment that you start your talk, and you are convinced that everyone thinks you are stupid.

> ✔ You realise that your fear is greater than the situation really warrants. For example, if you fear meeting new people, logically you know that nothing horrible will happen, but tidal waves of adrenaline course through your veins, and fearful anticipation threatens to overwhelm you.

> ✔ You avoid fearful situations as much as you can or endure them only with great distress.

Read the following prime example of a social phobic and see whether any of it seems familiar.

Paul, a 35-year-old eligible bachelor, really wants a serious, long-term relationship. Women consider him fairly attractive, he dresses well, and he has a very good, well-paid job. Paul's friends invite him to parties and other social events in an effort to matchmake. Unfortunately, he detests the idea of going. His latest invitation is for a New Year's party. On Boxing Day, he starts dreading the party. In his mind, Paul conjures up a number of good excuses for backing out. However, his desire to meet potential partners eventually wins. He runs scenes of meeting women over and over in his mind. Each time that he imagines one of these scenes, he feels intense, anxious anticipation. He berates himself, knowing at one level that his fear is ridiculous but feeling powerless to do anything about it.

On the day of the party, he has no appetite and barely eats a thing. Then he spends hours getting ready, casting aside outfit after outfit, feeling that nothing suits him. When Paul arrives at the party, he heads straight for the bar to drown his mounting anxiety. His hands shake as he picks up his first drink. Quickly downing the drink, he orders another, trying to calm himself. After an hour of non-stop drinking, he feels much braver. He interrupts a cluster of attractive women and comes out with a string of jokes that he's memorised for the occasion. They all fall flat. Then he approaches various women throughout the night, sometimes making flirtatious, suggestive comments. He doesn't get far, but he feels good about his performance.

The next day, Paul awakens in an unfamiliar bedroom, not remembering the end of the evening. His friend looks into the room and says, 'You were so far gone last night that we took your keys and put you to bed. Do you remember what happened?' Paul shakes his head, his face flushed with embarrassment. His friend continues, 'Well, I hate to tell you this, but you were making some pretty raunchy approaches to Brenda. She got quite upset. Her brother almost lost it with you, and you were quite ready to have a go at him. All in all, it wasn't a pretty sight.'

Paul has social phobia. Drug and alcohol abuse often accompany social phobia. Perhaps you can see why.

Feeling panicky

Of course, everyone feels some panic from time to time. People often say that they're panicking about a looming deadline or a presentation, or about planning a party. You're likely to hear the term used to describe concerns about rather mundane events such as these.

But people who suffer with panic disorders are talking about different phenomena entirely. They have periods of horrendously intense fear and anxiety. If you've never had a panic attack, you're lucky. The attacks usually last about ten minutes, and many people who have them really believe that they will die during the attack. Not exactly the best ten minutes of their lives. Panic attacks normally include a range of attention-grabbing symptoms, such as:

- Irregular, rapid, or pounding heartbeat
- Perspiring
- A sense of choking, suffocation, or shortness of breath
- Vertigo or light-headedness
- Pain or other discomfort in your chest
- Feeling that events are unreal or a sense of detachment from yourself
- Numbness or tingling
- Hot or cold flashes
- Feeling that you will faint, have a heart attack, or a brain haemorrhage
- Fearing that you will die, though without basis in fact
- Stomach nausea or upset, or feeling that you will vomit
- Jitteriness or trembling
- Thoughts of going insane or completely losing control, or of making a fool of yourself
- Feeling that you will lose control of your bladder or bowels, or both

Professionals generally agree that in order to have full-blown panic disorder, panic attacks must occur more than once. People with panic disorder worry about when they'll experience the next attack and whether they'll lose control and/or embarrass themselves. Finally, they usually start changing their lives by avoiding certain places or activities.

Panic attacks often begin with an event, such as physical exertion or normal variations in the body's reactions, that triggers some kind of sensation. This triggering event induces responses in the body, such as increased levels of adrenaline. No problem so far.

But the otherwise-normal process goes awry at the next step – when the person who suffers from panic attacks then misinterprets the meaning of the physical symptoms. Rather than viewing the symptoms as normal, the person with panic disorder sees them as a signal that something dangerous is happening, such as a heart attack, brain haemorrhage, or a stroke. That interpretation causes escalating fear and thus more physical arousal. In other words, it becomes a vicious cycle. Fortunately, the body sustains such heightened physical responses only for a while, and it eventually calms down.

The good news: Many people have a single panic attack and never have another one. So don't panic if you have a panic attack.

Maria's story is a good example of a one-off panic attack.

Maria leaves the hospital after visiting her next-door neighbour. She still can't believe that he had a heart attack at the age of 42. Maria, never one to worry about her health, ponders the fact that she just reached her 46th birthday. She resolves to lose that extra stone or so and to start exercising.

On her third visit to the gym, frustrated with her slow progress, she sets the treadmill to level 6. Almost immediately, her heart rate accelerates rapidly. Alarmed, she decreases the level to 3. She starts taking rapid, shallow breaths but feels she can't get enough air. Reducing the level further doesn't seem to help. She stops the treadmill and goes to the changing room. Sweating profusely and feeling nauseous, she finds an empty cubicle. She sits down and thinks that maybe she just overdid the treadmill a little. But the symptoms intensify and her chest tightens. She wants to scream but feels she can't get enough air. She's sure that she'll pass out and hopes someone will find her before she dies. She hears someone pass by and weakly calls for help. An ambulance whisks her to the nearest casualty department while she prays that she'll live through her heart attack.

In casualty, Maria's symptoms subside, and the doctor comes in to explain the results of her examination. He says that she's apparently experienced a panic attack and enquires about what may have triggered it. She explains that she was exercising due to concerns about her weight and health, and she mentions her neighbour's heart attack.

'Ah ha!' says the doctor reassuringly. 'Your health worries made you hypersensitive to any bodily symptom. When your heart rate naturally increased on the treadmill, you became frightened. That fear caused your body to produce more adrenaline, which in turn created more symptoms, including an increase in heart rate. The more symptoms you had, the more your fear and adrenaline increased. If you understand this, hopefully, in the future, your body's normal physical variations won't frighten you. Your heart's in great shape. I recommend that you go back to exercising but just increase it slowly over time without sudden jumps in intensity. Also, you may try some simple relaxation techniques; I'll ask the nurse to come in and tell you about those. I have every reason to believe that you won't have another episode like this one. Finally, you may want to read *Overcoming Anxiety For Dummies* by Elaine Iljon Foreman, Charles Elliott, and Laura Smith (Wiley); it's a great book!'

Maria doesn't have a diagnosis of panic disorder because she hasn't experienced more than one attack and she may never have another panic attack again. If she believes the doctor and takes his advice, the next time that her heart races, she probably won't get so scared. She may even use the relaxation techniques that the nurse explained to her – or even the others she picked up from the book!

If you worry that you have panic disorder, remember that it can be treated. This chapter gives you the knowledge that you need, and other chapters (see especially Chapters 8 and 10) tell you how to combine your understanding with actions.

The panic companion – agoraphobia

Around half of those with panic disorder have an accompanying problem: *agoraphobia*. The word comes from the Greek *agora,* meaning marketplace, and *phobia* – well you know that one by now. Any open space, whether a beach, a field, or a sports stadium, can leave the person paralysed with terror. However, agoraphobia is not just a fear of open spaces; the real underlying fear is more complex, encompassing several aspects of daily life that are closely interlinked. The phobias or fears in agoraphobia involve activities such as leaving home, entering public places, or travelling alone. In these situations the person feels especially vulnerable and exposed, with nowhere to escape to or hide if things go wrong. Agoraphobia therefore often includes fear of visiting supermarkets or going to the theatre or cinema.

Unlike most fears or phobias, this disorder usually begins in adulthood. Individuals with agoraphobia live in terror of feeling overwhelmed by panic. In addition, they worry about what will happen to them if they have a panic attack. They desperately avoid situations from which they can't readily escape, and they also fear places where help may not be readily forthcoming should they need it. The agoraphobic may start with one fear, such as being in a crowd, but in many cases the feared situations multiply to the point that the person fears even leaving home. And the last straw for some people is that they then start to worry 'What if I have one of my "funny turns" when I'm at home alone, with no-one to help me?' So even home is no longer a sanctuary.

Help! I'm dying!

Panic attack symptoms, such as chest pain, shortness of breath, nausea, and intense fear, often resemble those of heart attacks. Alarmed, those who experience these terrifying episodes head for the nearest casualty department. Then after numerous tests come back negative, overworked doctors tell the victim of a panic attack in so many words, 'It's all in your mind.' Unbelieving panic attack patients are sure that the doctor must have missed something. The next time they have a panic attack, they are likely to return to casualty for another opinion, doing this again and again. The repeat visits frustrate people with panic attacks as well as the hospital staff. However, a simple 20- or 30-minute psychological intervention in the casualty department decreases the repeat visits dramatically. What is the intervention? It can be just providing education about what the disorder is all about and describing a few deep relaxation techniques to try out when panic attacks strike. It certainly made a difference to Maria. (You'll find many more ideas in this book; read on.)

When agoraphobia combines with panic disorder, individuals fear any situation in which they may have an attack. As agoraphobia teams up with panic, the double-barrelled fear of not getting help, and horror at the idea of feeling overwhelmed and unable to control the feelings, frequently lead to paralysing isolation.

You or someone you love may have agoraphobia if

- ✔ You worry about being somewhere where you can't easily leave or can't get help if something 'terrible' happens, such as a panic attack.
- ✔ You tremble over everyday things, like leaving home, being in large groups of people, or travelling.
- ✔ Because of your anxiety, you avoid so much the places that you dread that your fear takes over your life and you become a prisoner of it.

You may have concerns about feeling trapped or have anxiety about crowds and leaving home. Many people do. But if your life goes on without major changes or constraints, you're probably not agoraphobic.

Nevertheless, you may still have problems with your fears in this area. For example, you may tremble at the thought of going to a live pop concert or large sporting event. You see images of stampeding crowds pushing and shoving, causing you to fall, only to be trampled by the mob as you cry out. If so, you may live an entire blissful life avoiding sports stadiums. Thus your fears don't bother you much. But if you love the atmosphere when watching live events, or perhaps you've just got a job as a reporter, this fear may be really bad news.

Patricia's story, which follows, demonstrates the overwhelming anxiety that often traps agoraphobics.

Patricia celebrates her 40th birthday without having experienced significant emotional problems. She's gone through the usual bumps in the road of life like losing a parent, her child having a learning disability, and a divorce ten years earlier. She prides herself on being able to cope with whatever cards life deals her.

Lately, she notices that she feels stressed when she goes shopping. She needs to pick up a birthday present and doesn't want to go because the shopping centre is especially crowded at weekends. She finally makes herself go to the shopping centre and finds a parking spot at the very end of a row. As she enters the shopping centre, heart pounding, her sweaty hands leave a smudge on the revolving glass door. She feels as though the crowds of shoppers are crushing her, and Patricia feels trapped. She's so scared that she can't bring herself to buy the present and flees the shopping centre.

Over the next few months, Patricia's fears spread. Although it started in the shopping centre, fear and anxiety now overwhelm her in any busy shop. Later, Patricia feels she can no longer cope when she's simply driving in traffic. Patricia is now suffering from agoraphobia. If not treated, Patricia may end up housebound.

Many times, panic, agoraphobia, and anxiety strike people who are otherwise devoid of serious, deep-seated emotional problems. So if you suffer from anxiety, it doesn't necessarily mean you'll need years of psychotherapy. You may not like the anxiety, but you certainly don't have to put up with it!

Specific phobias – spiders, snakes, lightning, planes, and other scary things

Many fears appear to be almost hard-wired into the human brain, they're so common. Cavemen and women had good reasons to fear snakes, strangers, heights, darkness, open spaces, and the sight of blood: Snakes could be poisonous, strangers could be enemies, a person could fall from a height, darkness could harbour unknown hazards, open spaces could leave a primitive tribe vulnerable to attack from all sides, and the sight of blood could signal a crisis, even potential death. Throwing up could be a warning to stop eating immediately – were those mushrooms edible or poisonous? Fear inspired caution and avoidance of harm. Those with these fears had a better chance of survival than the naively brave.

That's why many of the most common fears today reflect the dangers of the world thousands of years ago. Even today, it makes sense to cautiously identify a spider before you pick it up. However, sometimes fears rise to a disabling level. You may have a specific phobia if

- ✔ You have an exaggerated fear of a specific situation or object.

- ✔ When you're in fearful situations, you experience excessive anxiety immediately. Your anxiety may include sweating, rapid heartbeat, a desire to flee, tightness in the chest or throat, or images of something awful happening.

- ✔ You know that the fear is unreasonable. However, a child with a specific phobia doesn't always know that the phobia is unreasonable. For example, the child may really think that *all* dogs bite.

- ✔ You avoid your feared object or situation as much as you possibly can.

- ✔ Because your fear is so intense, you go so far as to change your day-to-day behaviour at work, at home, or in relationships. Thus, your fear inconveniences you and perhaps others, and it restricts your life.

Almost two-thirds of people fear one thing or another. For example, Laura Smith (one of the authors of this book), hates bugs. She says, 'Whenever a cricket is in the house, I avoid it or get someone else to dispose of it. One year, I had an office in an old building. Every morning, dead cockroaches littered the floor. I devised ways of getting them out of my office using a huge wad of paper towels. If instead I had quit my job because of the bugs, I would have had a diagnosis of specific phobia. But my fears don't significantly interfere with my life. You, like me, may have an excessive fear of something. That doesn't mean that you have a specific phobia in the diagnosable sense, as long as it doesn't disrupt your life in a major way. And you may or may not want to do something about it. In case you're wondering, I don't particularly mind the fact that bugs gross me out; I intend to live out my entire life in this manner and have no desire to work on this problem.'

The following description of Ted's life gives a typical picture of what someone with a specific phobia goes through.

Ted trudges up eight flights of stairs each morning to get to his office and tells everyone that he loves the exercise. When Ted passes the lift on the way to the stairs, his heart pounds, and he feels a sense of doom. Ted envisions being trapped in the lift – the doors close and there's no escape. In his mind, the lift rises on rusty cables, makes sudden jerks up and down, then goes into freefall and crashes into the basement.

Ted has never experienced anything like his fantasy, nor has anyone he knows had this experience. He never liked lifts, but didn't start avoiding them until the past few years. It seems that the more he avoids using them, the stronger his fear grows. He used to feel okay on escalators, but now he finds himself avoiding those as well. Several weeks ago, at the airport, he had no alternative but to take the escalator. He managed to get on, but became so frightened that he had to sit down for a while after he reached the second floor.

One afternoon, Ted rushes down the stairs after work, running late for an appointment. He slips and falls, breaking his leg. Now in a cast, with eight flights of stairs no longer an option, Ted faces the challenge of his life. Ted has a specific phobia.

Post-traumatic stress disorder: Feeling the aftermath

Tragically, war, rape, terror, serious accidents, brutality, torture, and natural disasters can be a part of life. You or someone you know may have experienced one of life's traumas. No-one knows why for sure, but some people seem to recover from these events without disabling symptoms. However, many others suffer considerably after their tragedies, sometimes for a lifetime.

More often than not, trauma causes at least a few uncomfortable emotional and/or physical reactions for a while. These responses can show up immediately after the disaster, or sometimes they emerge years later. These symptoms are the way that the body and mind deal with and process what happened. If an extremely unfortunate event occurs, it's normal to react strongly.

Top ten fears

Various polls and surveys collect information about what people fear most. In the following list, we compile the most common fears. Do you have any of these?

10 Dogs

 9 Being alone at night

 8 Thunder and lightning

 7 Spiders and insects

 6 Being trapped in a small space

 5 Flying

 4 Rodents

 3 Heights

 2 Giving a speech

And finally, the number one fear: Snakes

The diagnosis of *post-traumatic stress disorder* (PTSD) is complicated. If you suspect that you may have it, you should seek professional help. On the other hand, you may realise that you have a few of these symptoms but not the full diagnosis. If so, and if your problem feels mild and doesn't interfere with your life, you may want to try working on the difficulty on your own for a while. But seek help if you don't feel better.

The way in which reactions can arise years later (delayed PTSD) is illustrated by what happens to **James.** He seeks help, troubled by nightmares, sleep disturbance, irritability, and a whole host of unhappy feelings. Sometimes an image pops into his head – a small spark from a wire that he had known shouldn't be live. This makes no sense, and he thinks that he must be going crazy. Turns out, many years before, he'd suffered near electrocution from a live Underground rail he'd been working on, which was supposed to have no current. But at that time, he just got on with his work and life and had no symptoms at all. Then the little spark – and all the reactions to the major traumatic event – surfaced for the first time, and James found himself suffering from full-blown PTSD.

You may have PTSD if you personally experienced or witnessed an event that you perceived as potentially life threatening or causing serious injury, or you discovered that someone close to you experienced such an event. If your response to such an event includes terror, horror, or helplessness, you may develop PTSD, and you may also experience the following three types of problems:

- ✔ You *relive* the event in one or more of the ways shown in the following examples:

  - Having unwanted memories or flashbacks during the day or in your dreams

  - Feeling the trauma is happening again

  - Experiencing physical or emotional reactions when reminded of the event

- ✔ You *avoid* anything that reminds you of the trauma and try to suppress or numb your feelings in several ways. These include:

  - Trying to block out thinking or talking about the event because you get upset when you remember what happened

  - Staying away from people or places that remind you of the trauma

  - Losing interest in life or feeling distant from people

  - Sensing somehow that you don't have a long future

  - Feeling numb or detached

✔ You feel *on guard and stirred up* in several ways. Examples of this are:

- Becoming startled more easily
- Losing your temper quickly and feeling irritable
- Failing to concentrate as well as before
- Sleeping fitfully

What's it like to live with PTSD? For Charles, it's a constant struggle.

Charles is a colonel in the army. Since the first Gulf War, things have been a struggle for Charles. He sleeps poorly and has frequent nightmares; he loses his temper easily, and he feels detached from life.

Charles assumes his problems all stem from issues relating to the army: his work hours, frequent separations from his family, and numerous transfers, which mean moving house frequently, all the while with the intense pressure for promotion. He looks forward to retirement and a less stressful lifestyle. He promises his wife and children that his first goal on retirement is to spend more time with them.

But when Charles takes early retirement at 50, he finds it less rewarding than he'd hoped. He continues to have trouble sleeping. He tries to fulfil his promise to his family but just can't muster any enthusiasm for their activities. He doesn't find anything to look forward to, and his distance from his family grows. He continues to feel irritable and jumpy. After six months of retirement, Charles's wife insists they go for marital counselling.

In taking their history, the psychologist asks Charles about his Gulf War experience. Charles replies shortly that he doesn't want to talk about it – that's how he handles the disturbing memories of the war. That unwillingness to discuss it, together with Charles' other problems, suggests to the psychologist that Charles may have PTSD.

Obsessive-compulsive disorder – over and over and over again

Obsessive-compulsive disorder (OCD) wreaks incredible havoc on people's lives, because OCD frequently frustrates and confuses not only the people afflicted with it, but also their families and loved ones. If untreated, OCD is likely to last a lifetime. Even with treatment, symptoms often recur. That's the bad news. Thankfully, effective treatments are available. So even if the problem comes back, which it may on more than one occasion, you have the skills to deal with it.

A person with OCD may exhibit behaviours that include obsessional thoughts or compulsions, or both. So what are obsessions versus compulsions?

Obsessions are unwelcome repetitive images, impulses, or thoughts that come into your mind. People find these thoughts and images disturbing and can't get rid of them. For example, a religious man may have a thought that he will start shouting obscenities during a church service, or a caring mother may have intrusive thoughts of causing harm to her baby. While the vast majority of people don't carry out these imagined actions, the obsessions still haunt them.

Compulsions are undesired repetitive actions or mental strategies carried out to temporarily reduce anxiety. From time to time, an obsessional thought triggers the anxiety; at other times, the anxiety may be triggered by an obsessional thought or a feared event or situation.

For example, **Mary** washes her hands literally hundreds of times each day or feels compelled to wash them a certain number of times, or in a certain way, in order to reduce her anxiety about germs. **Ally** has an elaborate night-time ritual of touching certain objects, lining up clothes in a specific way, arranging his wallet next to the house keys in a special position, stacking loose change, getting into bed in precisely the correct manner, and reading one section of the Bible before turning out the light. And if either Mary or Ally performs any part of the ritual in less than the 'perfect' way, she or he feels compelled to start all over until it is right. They have the awful feeling that something terrible will befall them or their loved ones if they fail to get it right.

You may have obsessive-compulsive disorder (OCD) if you have obsessions, compulsions, or both. *Obsessions* work like this:

✔ **Your obsessional thoughts do not involve real-life problems.**

For example, if you worry about germs on your hands and you're a brain surgeon, we're glad about that, and you're being realistic. But if you constantly worry about germs on your hands and you work in a library, you just may have an obsessional problem.

✔ **When the thoughts occur, you try to get rid of them by thinking or doing something else.**

For example, you may have a special prayer or saying that you repeat in your mind over and over again.

✔ **You know that your obsessional thoughts are coming from your own mind and not from some other source.**

If you do feel that someone or something is putting thoughts into your head, then this is a different type of problem to OCD and you should get professional help for it.

✔ **The thoughts bother you considerably.**

You try to banish the thoughts, but invariably they return and are very upsetting and distressing.

The following applies to *compulsions:*

✔ Compulsions are actions and behaviours or mental strategies that you feel compelled to repeat again and again in response to one of your obsessional thoughts or because you have a belief in some rigid rule that you feel can't be broken.

✔ You believe that your compulsive acts can in some way prevent a terrible event from happening, or that they are the only way to alleviate your anxiety, but you are aware that what you do doesn't really make much sense.

The OCD cycle

A pattern frequently develops in which obsessional thoughts create anxiety, which causes the person to engage in a compulsive act in order to reduce the anxiety and obtain relief. That temporary relief powerfully encourages the person to believe that the compulsive act helps. Unfortunately, the cycle begins again, because the obsessional thoughts return. Table 2-1 shows common thoughts and the behaviours which often follow.

Table 2-1   The Most Common Obsessions and Compulsions

Obsessions	*Compulsions*
Worry about contamination, such as from dirt, germs, radiation, and chemicals.	Excessive hand-washing or cleaning due to the obsessive fear of contamination.
Doubts about having remembered to turn the cooker and the lights off, lock the doors, close the windows, and so on.	Checking and rechecking to see that the cooker is off, doors and windows are locked, and so on. Even returning home after leaving to re-check.
Sexual imagery about which you feel ashamed.	Repeating certain words or phrases to stop yourself acting on disturbing thoughts – though you never have acted them out.
Thoughts that would violate your own personal codes of behaviour in some shameful way.	Arranging items in a rigid, precise way. Often, you feel compelled to start again if it doesn't come out perfectly.
Thoughts urging you to behave in a socially strange and unacceptable way.	Preventative behaviours such as counting stairs, ceiling tiles, steps walked, and so on. Can include repeating actions such as walking back and forth through a doorway until 'good thoughts' accompany you through the doorway.

(continued)

Table 2-1 *(continued)*

Obsessions	Compulsions
Unwanted thoughts of harming someone you love.	Repeating rituals over and over again, with a belief that this will somehow prevent something bad from happening. The belief is that the ritual must be carried out correctly for it to be effective.
Fears of harming others.	Avoiding using knives even when cooking. Not holding or playing with young children. Repeatedly driving back over your route to check you haven't run someone over. (And then having to drive the route again to check out that journey.) Moving stones and objects off footpaths to stop others tripping – and then worrying that the new placement will cause an accident.

Seeing OCD when it's not there

You may recall walking to school with your friends and avoiding cracks in the pavement. If you accidentally stepped on one, perhaps someone scolded, 'If you step on a crack, you'll break your mother's back!' And perhaps sometimes you walked to school by yourself, and that same thought occurred to you, so you avoided stepping on the cracks. Obviously you knew that stepping on a crack wouldn't break your mother's back, so not stepping on cracks doesn't really qualify as a compulsion – even if you did it repeatedly – if you knew it wouldn't stop anything bad from happening. If you did it simply as a game and it didn't bother you that much, avoiding cracks was no big deal. As we all know, kids often have magical or superstitious thinking, which they usually outgrow.

On the other hand, if some part of you really worried that your mother may suffer if you stepped on a crack, and if you couldn't even get to school because of your worry, you probably had full-blown compulsive behaviour. Many people check the locks more than once, go back a few times to make sure that the oven is turned off, or count stairs or steps unnecessarily. It's only when doing these things starts taking too much time and interferes with relationships, work, or everyday life that you really have a problem.

Lisa's extreme preoccupation with hanging on to objects of no value that only clutter up her home is an example of someone with OCD. Lisa is a collector, but you can't really call her a collector in the way most people think about collecting, because what she accumulates never has any real value to anyone. She is really a *hoarder*. She keeps every supermarket plastic bag and never

Avoiding anxiety only worsens anxiety

Avoidance underlies all the anxiety disorders. No-one likes to feel anxious. People generally respond to anxiety by steering clear of the things that make them anxious. It makes sense, doesn't it?

Well, yes and no. At the moment of avoidance, anxiety decreases. The problem is that the momentary relief actually increases the desire to continue avoiding the situation. Furthermore, the range of feared events starts to increase. Check out the following example:

Alan is a teacher. His wife has just left him, after Alan discovered that she had been having an affair with his best friend. He throws himself deeper into his work. Then one day he gets a thought – 'What if I were to expose myself to the two girls in the class I have booked for detention this evening?' He is horrified at this thought. However, he tells himself that the fact that he has had it means that he may really do it, even against his will. So he cancels the detention, feigning illness as the excuse. And feels a huge sense of relief.

But classroom control becomes an issue, as he can no longer use detention as a deterrent and punishment for bad behaviour. Thoughts of the 'What if?' type increasingly play on his mind, and he loses concentration during lessons. And the more he tells himself 'DON'T THINK ABOUT IT!', the more intrusive the thoughts become. He worries that if this has happened at school, should he be careful around his young niece? So he starts making excuses and cuts himself off from his sister's family, losing the support he needs at a time of isolation and the break-up of his marriage. Eventually, Alan goes to see his doctor, and is signed off work with obsessive compulsive disorder. His GP then refers him to the new primary mental health team – or the community mental health team – for psychological therapy.

That's how avoidance works. Avoidance feeds your fears. With enough avoidance, anxiety grows out of control.

Everyone avoids a few things. You may avoid snakes, and it's no big deal because they're pretty easy to avoid. You may even avoid an occasional social gathering that makes you anxious. As long as you can go to at least some social gatherings, your anxiety isn't likely to grow.

---

throws away a newspaper or magazine. Her garage holds nothing but a hotch-potch of batteries (most long out of date), string, bits of wire, nuts and bolts, and scraps of paper. Lisa simply can't get herself to throw anything away. Her house bursts at the seams with useless junk.

But Lisa thinks that just maybe one day that she may need some of these items, and she cannot decide what to keep and what to throw away. When she does think of something she needs, she can rarely find it in all the piles of rubble. As the years go by, Lisa becomes isolated. She can't invite anyone over, because she is embarrassed by the way her house looks. All the rooms are piled with bags of stuff, and she worries about the fire hazard and her family tripping up on the piles. Lisa's obsession centres around having something she needs. Thus she has a compulsion to never throw anything out. Lisa suffers from OCD.

Sorting Out What's Normal from What's Not

Imagine a life with no anxiety at all. How wonderful. You awaken every morning anticipating nothing but pleasant experiences. You fear nothing. The future holds only sweet security and joy.

Think again. With no anxiety, when the driver of the car in front of you slams on the brakes, your response is slower, and you'll crash. With no worries about the future, your retirement may end up bleak. The total absence of anxiety may mean you arrive unprepared for a work presentation.

Anxiety is good for you! It prepares you to take action. It mobilises your body for emergencies. It warns you about potential problems. Be glad you have some anxiety. Your anxiety helps you stay out of trouble.

Anxiety only poses a problem for you when

- ✔ Anxiety lasts uncomfortably long or occurs too often.
- ✔ It interferes with doing what you want to do.
- ✔ Anxiety greatly exceeds the level of actual danger or risk. For example, when your body and mind feel like an avalanche is about to bury you, but all you have to do is take a test at school, your anxiety has gone too far.
- ✔ You struggle to control your worries, but they keep disturbing you and never let up.

Knowing What Anxiety Isn't

Anxious symptoms may travel with other company. Thus you may have anxiety along with other emotional disorders. In fact, about half of those with anxiety disorders develop depression, especially if their anxiety goes untreated. The treatment of other emotional problems differs somewhat from the treatment of anxiety. So knowing the difference between those problems and anxiety is important. Of course, people have both sometimes.

In addition, medication effects and medical conditions can cause symptoms similar to those of anxiety. You may think that you're terribly anxious, but actually you may be physically ill or suffering from the side effects of a drug.

Beyond anxiety disorders

We want you to know that if you have anxiety, it means nothing about whether you have one of these other disorders. So realise that anxiety by itself is not one of these problems:

- **Depression:** Depression can make you feel like you're living life in slow motion. You lose interest in activities that used to bring you pleasure. You feel sad. Most likely, you feel tired, and you sleep fitfully. Your appetite may wane, and your sex drive may drop. The future looks bleak. As with anxiety, you may find it difficult to concentrate or plan ahead. But unlike anxiety, depression saps your drive and motivation.

- **Bipolar disorder, or manic depression:** With this disorder, your mood seesaws between ups and downs. At times, you feel that you're on top of the world. You have grandiose ideas and need little sleep. You may invest in risky schemes, shop recklessly, engage in sexual escapades, or lose your good judgement in other ways. You may start working frantically on important projects or find ideas streaming through your mind. Then suddenly your mood goes crashing downward, and you find yourself experiencing depression.

- **Schizophrenia:** This type of psychotic disorder may make you feel anxious, but the symptoms profoundly disrupt life. It can weave hallucinations into everyday life. For example, some people hear voices talking to them or see shadowy figures when no-one is around. Delusions, another feature, also distort reality. Common psychotic delusions include believing that MI5 or aliens are tracking your whereabouts, or that people close to you mean you harm. Other delusions involve grandiose beliefs, such as thinking that you're Jesus Christ or that you have a special mission to save the world.

  If you think that you hear the phone ringing when you're drying your hair or in the shower, only to discover that it wasn't, you're not suffering from psychosis. Most people occasionally hear or see trivial things that aren't there. It's only when these perceptions seriously depart from reality that this may be one of the psychotic disorders, and you should seek professional help. It's important to realise that anxiety disorders don't lead to psychosis.

- **Substance abuse:** When people develop a dependency on drugs or alcohol, withdrawal may create serious anxiety. The symptoms of drug or alcohol withdrawal include tremors, disrupted sleep, sweating, increased heartbeat, agitation, and tension. However, if these symptoms only come on in response to a recent cessation of substance use, it's not an anxiety disorder. On the other hand, those with anxiety disorders sometimes abuse substances in the misguided attempt to control their anxiety.

Mimicking Anxiety: Drugs and Diseases

As common as anxiety disorders are, believing that you're suffering from anxiety when you're not is all too easy. Prescription drugs may have a variety of side effects, some of which mimic some of the symptoms of anxiety. Various medical conditions also produce symptoms that imitate the signs of anxiety.

Exploring anxiety-mimicking drugs

The pharmaceutical industry reports on the most widely prescribed categories of medications every year. Some drugs which can have anxiety-mimicking side effects are:

- Alcohol
- Caffeine
- Illegal drugs, such as amphetamines, cocaine, cannabis, ecstasy, and LSD
- Some antidepressants such as fluoxetine and paroxetine
- Salbutamol inhalers for asthma, if used too much
- Steroids, such asprednisolone or dexamethasone in higher doses
- Thyroxine, if the dose is too high
- Insulin, if the dose is too high
- Digoxin, if the dose is too high or the patient becomes dehydrated
- Lithium-based mood stabilisers when the dose is too high or the patient becomes dehydrated
- Slimming pills

Interesting isn't it? Even medications used for the treatment of anxiety, such as some mood stabilisers and antidepressants, can produce anxiety-like side effects. Of course, most people don't experience such side effects with these medications, but they do occur. If you're taking one or more of the commonly prescribed or over-the-counter medications in this list and feel anxious, you may want to check with your doctor.

Angst from over the counter

One of the most common ingredients in over-the-counter cold medications is *pseudoephedrine,* a popular and effective decongestant. Charles Elliott (one of the team writing this book) specialises in the treatment of panic and anxiety disorders. He says, 'A couple of years ago, I had a bad cold and cough for longer than usual. I treated it with the strongest over-the-counter medications that I could find. Not only that, I took a little more than the label called for during the day, so I could see clients without coughing through the session. One day during that period, I noticed an unusually rapid heartbeat and considerable tightness in breathing. I wondered for

a while whether I was having a panic attack. It didn't seem possible, but the symptoms stared me in the face. Could I possibly have caught panic disorder from my clients?

Not exactly. Upon reflection, I realised that perhaps I'd taken more than just a little too much of the cold medication containing pseudoephedrine. I stopped taking the medication, and the symptoms disappeared, never to return.

So be careful with over-the-counter medications. Read the directions carefully. Don't try to be your own doctor like I did!'

Investigating medical conditions with accompanying anxiety

More than a few types of diseases and medical conditions can create anxiety-like symptoms. That's why we strongly recommend, especially if you're experiencing significant anxiety for the first time, that you visit your doctor. Your doctor can help you sort out whether you have a physical problem, a reaction to medication, an emotionally based anxiety problem, or some combination of these.

Some problems arise suddenly and are short-lived, and these are called *acute* disorders. Problems that last longer and don't get better, sometimes without and sometimes even with treatment, are called *chronic* disorders.

Table 2-2 lists some of the medical conditions that produce anxiety symptoms. In addition, merely getting sick can cause anxiety about your illness. For example, if you receive a serious diagnosis of heart disease, cancer, or a chronic progressive disorder, you are likely to develop some anxiety about dealing with the consequences of what you've been told. The same techniques for dealing with anxiety throughout this book can help you with this type of anxiety as well.

Table 2-2	Medical Mimics	
Medical Condition	*What It Is*	*Anxiety-like Symptoms*
Hypoglycaemia	Low blood sugar, associated with other disorders or occuring by itself. It is a common complication of diabetes.	Confusion, irritability, trembling, sweating, rapid heartbeat, weakness, and a cold clammy feeling.
Hyperthyroidism	Excess amount of thyroid hormone. It has various causes.	Nervousness, restlessness, sweating, fatigue, sleep disturbance, nausea, tremor, and diarrhoea.
Other hormonal imbalances	Various events and conditions associated with fluctuations in hormone levels, such as premenstrual syndrome (PMS), menopause, or childbirth. Highly variable symptoms.	Tension, irritability, headaches, mood swings, compulsive behaviour, fatigue, and panic.
Heart arrhythmias	Mainly in the elderly or people with heart disease, and sometimes in alcoholics, the heart can start to beat irregularly. This is called a trial fibrillation. If this is very fast then it can cause symptoms that resemble anxiety.	Palpitations, shortness of breath, fatigue, chest pain, and difficulty breathing.
Ménière's syndrome	An inner-ear disorder, caused by pressure exerted by excess fluid in the inner ear.	Vertigo that includes abnormal sensations associated with movement, dizziness, nausea, vomiting, and sweating.

Stress and Health

If we perceive events to be a threat to our normal functioning, wellbeing, or self-esteem, we experience the negative thoughts and emotions we all associate with stress. However, the effects of stress are not limited to what goes on within our brains – they permeate our whole body and, if sustained, can have powerful and harmful effects on our physical health. It's the link between what we think or feel and the activity in the rest of our body that's mediated (at least in part) by the stress hormone *cortisol*. The more stressful we perceive life to be, the more cortisol is released into the bloodstream. Although cortisol is an essential hormone that performs a wide range of vital functions (see "Understanding how cortisol works" later in this chapter), producing too much at the wrong times of day can put our health at risk.

The reason why the links between stress and health are so difficult to prove is because stress, and stress alone, does not cause a specific disease. Rather, a sustained period of stress can increase our chances of succumbing to a range of illnesses, depending on individual susceptibilities in terms of genetic predisposition and lifestyle. Potentially, stress can also worsen some existing conditions. Although it can be difficult to tease out all the factors that may lead to illness, research continues to find clear evidence that stress is an issue we should all take seriously: Stress not only threatens the quality of our lives but also the state of our health.

Understanding how cortisol works

Healthy levels of cortisol rise sharply within the first 30 minutes after awakening in the morning and then decline throughout the rest of the day to reach their lowest levels before going to bed and in the early stages of sleep. This pattern is important as a 24-hour signal to the rest of the body, maintaining a healthy balance between the different organ systems during the course of the day. If too much stress is superimposed upon this normal, healthy pattern then the rest of the body doesn't know whether it's night or day, and this can cause a problem for efficient functioning.

In addition, body organs detect stress-related increases in cortisol and respond in a variety of ways – for example, by increasing blood pressure, altering the balance of our immune systems, and increasing blood glucose levels for use as energy. Over-activity in any of these departments may increase the risk of cardiovascular problems, infection, and/or allergic disorders, as well as diabetes.

Preparing for fight or flight

Your body responds to threats by preparing for action in three different ways: physically, mentally, and behaviourally. When danger presents itself, you reflexively prepare to stand and fight or run like you've never run before. Your body mobilises to respond to danger in complex and fantastic ways.

Figure 2-1 gives you the picture.

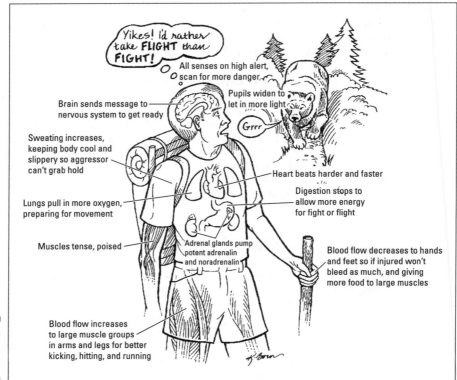

Figure 2-1:
Choices,
choices!

First, the brain sends signals through your nervous system for your body to go on high alert. Production and release of the stress hormone, cortisol, increases. The brain tells the adrenal glands to rev up production of adrenaline and noradrenaline. These hormones stimulate the body in various ways. Your heart pounds faster and faster, and you start breathing more rapidly, sending increased oxygen to your lungs, which is transferred to the blood that flows to the large muscles, preparing them to fight or flee from danger.

Digestion slows to preserve energy for meeting the challenge, and pupils dilate to improve vision. Blood flow decreases to hands and feet in order to prevent blood loss if injured and keep up the blood supply to the large muscles. Sweating increases in order to keep the body cool, and it makes you slippery, so aggressors can't grab hold of you. All your muscles tense to spring into action.

The chicken or the egg: Irritable bowel syndrome

Irritable bowel syndrome (IBS) is a common condition that involves a variety of related problems, usually including cramps or pain in the abdomen, diarrhoea, and/or constipation. These can occur in people with no known physical problems in their digestive systems. For many years, doctors told most of their patients that irritable bowel syndrome (IBS) was caused exclusively by stress, worry, and anxiety.

In 1999, Dr Catherine Woodman and colleagues discovered a mutated gene that occurred more often in patients with IBS than in those without IBS. Interestingly, that same rogue gene also occurs more often in those with panic disorders. Other possible physical causes of IBS may have to do with poor communication between muscles and nerves in the colon.

Various medications have been found to decrease some of the worst symptoms of IBS. In addition, psychological therapies such as cognitive behaviour therapy, plus relaxation techniques, biofeedback, and techniques for coping with anxiety and stress, also improve IBS symptoms. So at this point, no-one really knows how much IBS is due to physical causes, anxiety, or stress. However, studies have shown that long term perceived stress triples the rate of flare-ups compared with that in patients who did not report feelings of stress. It's therefore most likely that the mind and body interact in important ways that can't always be separated.

Mentally, you automatically scan your surroundings intensely. Your attention focuses on the threat and nothing else. In fact, you can't attend to much of anything else.

Behaviourally, you're now ready to flee or fight. You need that preparation in the face of danger. When you have to take on a bear, a lion, or a warrior, you'd better have all systems on high alert.

Just one problem – in today's world, most people don't encounter lions and bears. Unfortunately, your body doesn't know this and automatically reacts with the same preparation for facing dangers, even though these are fighting traffic, meeting deadlines, speaking in public, and other everyday worries.

When human beings have nothing to fight or run from, all that energy has to get out somehow. So you may feel the urge to fidget by moving your feet and hands. You feel on edge – like jumping out of your skin. You may be highly irritable with those around you.

Homing in on anxiety-related disorders

Most experts believe that if you experience these physical effects of anxiety on a frequent, chronic basis, it can't be doing you any good. Various studies have suggested the possibility that chronic anxiety and stress may conceivably contribute to a variety of physical problems, such as abnormal heart rhythms, high blood pressure, irritable bowel syndrome, asthma, ulcers, stomach upsets (diarrhoea, constipation, cramping, bloating, and excessive production of digestive acids in the stomach, which may cause a painful burning sensation), chronic muscle spasms, tremors, chronic back pain, tension, headaches (which may only start some time after the event), and a depressed immune system.

Figure 2-2 illustrates the toll of chronic anxiety on the body.

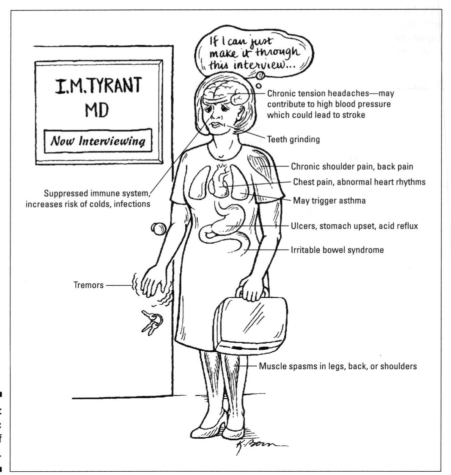

Figure 2-2:
The chronic effects of anxiety.

Chronic anxiety has also been implicated in:

- The development of depression
- The development of full-blown anxiety disorder
- Reduced quality of life by diminishing feelings of pleasure and accomplishment
- Potential damage to relationships
- Heart disease
- Stroke
- Effects on the inflammatory response
- Weight gain or loss
- Diabetes
- Sleep disturbances, including both insomnia and/or waking up in the middle of the night or early morning
- Diminished sexual desire and an inability to achieve orgasm in women
- Temporary impotence in men
- Negative effects on both fertility and pregnancy
- Memory, concentration, and learning disorders
- Allergies
  - eczema and other rashes
  - headaches
  - asthma
  - sinus problems
- Skin conditions, including
  - hives
  - psoriasis
  - acne
  - rosacea
  - eczema
  - unexplained itching
- Unexplained hair loss *(Alopecia areata):* where hair is lost in discrete patches. The cause is unknown, but stress is suspected as a player in this condition. For example, hair loss often occurs during periods of intense stress, such as grieving after a death.
- Gum disease leading to tooth loss.

Reasons to tackle stress

If just the misery of chronic anxiety isn't enough, another reason to work on getting rid of excess stress is that research shows that anxiety has a big part to play in physical illness. Take diabetes – people with long-lasting stress are significantly more likely to develop type 2 diabetes. This isn't surprising, because stress increases the levels of glucose in the bloodstream.

But relieving anxiety can relieve illness. Researchers at Duke University conducted a study with over 100 subjects and found that when stress management was added to the care of adults with diabetes, their blood sugar levels actually went down, as much as you would expect had the subjects been taking an extra diabetes-control drug. The stress management techniques weren't complex or time consuming. You can read about many of them in this book and try them for yourself.

Further research has shown that psychological stress can make you more susceptible to other illnesses as well, for instance viral infections. In the 1950s, Dr Thomas Holmes studied the relationship between emotions and disease, and in particular the association between stress and tuberculosis. He found that people who had experienced stressful situations, such as divorce, the death of a spouse, or loss of a job, were more likely to develop tuberculosis and less likely to recover from it. Holmes emphasised the need to understand each patient's story and to view his or her tuberculosis as the culmination of a life of emotional hardship. Recent research supports Holmes's findings, suggesting that stress may lead to decreased immune function and thus to clinical disease.

Finally, numerous studies with patients undergoing life-threatening diseases such as AIDS suggest that those who remain optimistic show symptoms later and survive longer than those who confront reality more objectively. Optimistic patients are more likely to practise habits that enhance health, and to enlist social support. It seems that positive thinking and combating anxiety are things you can do to help prevent and fight illness.

If stress becomes chronic, sufferers often experience loss of concentration at work and at home, and they may become inefficient and accident-prone. In children, the physiological responses to chronic stress can make learning difficult. Chronic stress in older people may also play an even more important role in memory loss than the aging process.

However, before you get too anxious about your anxiety, please realise that hard, definitive evidence doesn't exist yet to show that anxiety is a *major* cause of most of these problems. Nevertheless, enough studies have suggested that it can make these disorders worse and that you should probably take chronic anxiety seriously. In other words, be concerned, but DON'T PANIC!

Chapter 3

Overcoming Obstacles to Change

In This Chapter

▶ Finding out where your anxiety stems from

▶ Discovering that you're not to blame

▶ Understanding the reasons people resist change

▶ Jumping over obstacles

*T*he odds are that if you're reading this book, you want to do something about your own anxiety or help someone that you care about. If so, you should know that people start on the path to change with the best intentions, but as they move along, suddenly they encounter obstacles, and when the going gets tough, it's tough to keep going.

This chapter gives you ways to get round, over, under, or through those obstacles. First, we explain where anxiety comes from. When you understand the origins of anxiety, you can move from self-blame to self-acceptance, thus allowing you to redirect your energy towards more productive activities. Next, we show you the other large obstacles that can block the way to change. Finally, we give you effective strategies to keep you safe on the road to overcoming anxiety.

Unearthing the Roots of Anxiety

The three major causes of anxiety are

✔ **Genetics:** Your biological inheritance

✔ **Parenting:** The way that you were brought up

✔ **Trauma:** The horrifying events that can happen in life

Studies show that when people experience an unanticipated trauma, only a minority end up with severe anxiety. That's because anxiety usually stems from a combination of causes – perhaps genes and trauma, or trauma and parenting, or sometimes all three combine to induce anxiety. At the same time, just one factor, if formidable enough, can possibly cause the entire problem.

For example, **Gloria** grows up on a tough estate, where gangs and violence are commonplace, without developing terribly distressing symptoms. Even when she is mugged for her new mobile phone, she shows surprising resilience during her recovery. Surely she must have some robust, anti-anxiety genes and perhaps some pretty good parents as well in order to successfully endure such an experience. She moves away from the estate and thinks she has left the past behind her. However, she is then on a train going to work, and a gang come steaming through the train, robbing and threatening the passengers, Following this experience, Gloria develops serious problems with anxiety. She has sustained one trauma too many.

Thus you can never ascertain the exact cause of anyone's anxiety with absolute certainty. However, if you examine someone's childhood relationship with his or her parents, family history, and the various events in his or her life (such as accidents, war, disease, and so on), you can generally come up with some pretty good ideas as to why anxiety now causes problems. If you have anxiety, consider reviewing these possible causes of distress and think about which ones may have given you the most trouble.

But what difference does it make where your anxiety comes from? Overcoming anxiety doesn't absolutely require knowledge of where it originated. The remedies change little whether you were born with anxiety or acquired it much later in your life.

However, more quickly identifying the source of your anxiety can help you to realise that your anxiety isn't something that you brought on yourself. Anxiety develops for a number of good, solid reasons. The blame doesn't belong with the person who has anxiety.

Guilt and self-blame can only sap your energy. They drain resources and keep your focus away from the effort required for challenging your anxiety. By contrast, self-forgiveness and self-acceptance invigorate and vitalise your efforts.

Separating nature from nurture

If you suffer from excessive worries and tension, look around at the rest of your family. Of those who have an anxiety disorder, typically about a quarter of their relatives suffer with them. So your Uncle Ralph may not struggle with anxiety, though Aunt Belinda or your sister Charlotte just may.

Genetic culprits

In people with anxiety disorders, studies have found a genetic mutation that affects the availability of the brain's neurotransmitter *serotonin,* which is believed to contribute to emotional wellbeing. If you don't have enough serotonin floating around in your brain, you're likely to fall prey to worries, anxiety, or the blues. Medications can increase the availability of serotonin in the brain (see Chapter 15).

But you may argue that Uncle Ralph, Aunt Belinda, and your sister Charlotte all had to live with Nan, who'd make anyone anxious. In other words, they lived in an anxiety-inducing environment. Maybe it has nothing to do with their genes.

Various researchers have studied siblings and twins who live together to verify that genes do play an important role in how people experience and cope with anxiety. As predicted, identical twins were far more similar to each other in terms of anxiety than non-identical twins or other siblings. But even if you're born with a genetic predisposition towards anxiety, other factors such as environment, peers, and how your parents raised you enter into the mix.

It's my parents' fault!

Parent-bashing is in. Blaming parents for almost anything that ails you is easy. Parents usually do the best they can. Raising children poses a formidable task. So in most cases, parents don't deserve to be vilified. However, they do hold some responsibility for the way in which you were brought up and so may indeed have contributed to your woes.

Three parenting styles appear to foster anxiety in children:

- **Over-protective:** These parents shield their kids from every imaginable stress or harm. If their kids stumble, they try to swoop them up before they even hit the ground. When their kids get upset, they fix the problem. Not surprisingly, their kids fail to find out how to tolerate fear, anxiety, or frustration.

- **Over-controlling:** These parents micro-manage all their children's activities. They direct every detail from how they should play to what they should wear to how they solve arithmetical problems. They discourage independence and feed dependency and anxiety.

✔ **Inconsistent:** The parents in this group provide their kids with erratic rules and limits. One day, they respond with understanding when their kids have trouble with their homework; the next day, they explode when asked for help. These kids fail to discover the connection between their own efforts and a predictable outcome. Therefore, they feel that they have little control over what happens in life. It's no wonder they feel anxious.

It's the world's fault!

The world today moves at a faster pace than ever, and for many of us, the working week has got longer. Modern life is rife with both complexity and danger. Perhaps that's why mental health workers see so many people with anxiety-related problems. Four specific types of disturbing events can trigger a problem with anxiety even in someone who has never suffered from it much before:

✔ **Unanticipated threats:** Predictability and stability counteract anxiety, and the opposite fuels it. For example, **Ahmed** works long hours to make a decent living. Nevertheless, he just about manages from month to month, with little left for savings. An accidental slip on an icy pavement leaves him out of action for six weeks, and as he is self-employed, no money comes in. He now worries incessantly over his ability to pay bills. Even when he returns to work, he worries more than ever about the next financial disaster that awaits him.

✔ **Escalating demands:** Nothing is better than a promotion. At least that's what **Jake** thinks when his supervisor gives him a once-in-a-lifetime opportunity to direct the new high-risk research and development division at work. Jake never expected such a lofty position this early in his career, or the doubling of his salary. Of course, new duties, expectations, and responsibilities are part of the deal. Jake now begins to fret and worry. What if he fails to meet the challenge? Anxiety starts taking over his life.

✔ **Confidence killers: Tricia** is on top of the world. She has a good job and feels ecstatic about her forthcoming wedding. However, she is devastated when her fiancé breaks off the engagement. Now, she worries incessantly that something is wrong with her; perhaps she'll never have the life she envisioned for herself.

✔ **Terrorising trauma:** No-one ever wants to experience a horrifying or life-threatening experience. Unfortunately, these events do happen. Physical abuse, horrific accidents, battlefield injuries, and rape have occurred for centuries, and we suspect that they always will. When they do, severe problems with anxiety often emerge. (See Chapter 2 for information about post-traumatic stress disorder.)

Moving from Self-blame to Self-acceptance

Time and again, we see our worried, tense clients suffer from an additional, needless source of pain. Their anxiety is bad enough, but they also blame themselves *because* they have anxiety. If you do this to yourself, we suggest that you try Gary's approach to self-forgiveness and self-acceptance.

Gary developed panic disorder. His attacks of feeling nauseous, dizzy, out of breath, and thinking that he's going crazy have increased recently. He feels deep shame and embarrassment that someone like him has this problem. When he starts having panic attacks at work, he finally caves in and seeks help. He tells his psychologist that a real man would never have this kind of problem. His psychologist helps Gary to be more self-forgiving. He asks Gary to write down the three major causes of his anxiety. He guides him through thoroughly reviewing his life and asks him to come up with as many possible contributors to his worries as he can. Look at Table 3-1 in this chapter to see what Gary came up with.

Table 3-1	Gary's Anxiety Causes	
Possible Genetic Influence	*Parenting*	*Events: Old and New*
My Aunt Mary hardly ever leaves her house. Maybe she has the same problem I have.	Well, my father had quite an unpredictable temper. I never knew when he'd explode.	When I was six years old, we had a terrible car accident, and I spent three days in the hospital. I was scared.
My mother has always suffered from her nerves.	My mother's moods bounced all over the place. I could never tell how she'd react when I asked her for something.	My junior school was on a terrible estate. Gangs ruled. I had to look over my shoulder the whole time.
My cousin Margarita seems shy. Maybe she has too much anxiety.	My parents didn't do much socialising, as my mother got into such a state about entertaining.	My first marriage ended when I caught my wife being unfaithful. I couldn't believe that she would do something like that. Even though I trust my new wife, I worry too much about her faithfulness.

(continued)

Table 3-1 *(continued)*		
Possible Genetic Influence	*Parenting*	*Events: Old and New*
My brother worries all the time. He seems totally stressed.	My father always predicted the worst was going to happen.	Two years ago, I was diagnosed with diabetes. I worry too much about my health now.

If you'd like to better understand the causes of your anxiety, write them down like Gary did in Table 3-1. Create columns that are topped with the same headings – 'Possible Genetic Influence', 'Parenting', and 'Events: Old and New'. Take your time; don't rush it. You may write several drafts before you come up with a definitive list. You may want to do this task over several days.

After you list the likely culprits that led to your distress, ask yourself some questions like the ones that follow:

- Did I ask for my anxiety?
- Was there ever a time in my life when I actually wanted to feel anxious?
- Am I primarily to blame for my worries?
- What percentage of the blame can I realistically assign to myself as opposed to genes, parenting, and events, both old and new?
- If a couple of friends of mine had trouble with anxiety, what would I say to them?
  - Would I think that they were to blame?
  - Would I think as badly of them as I do of myself?
- Does thinking badly about myself help me get over my anxiety?
- If I decided to stop beating myself up, would I have more energy for tackling my problems?

Hopefully, these questions can help you move towards self-acceptance. When you discover that having anxiety means nothing about your worth as a human being, you just may go a bit easier on yourself. We recommend it highly. If you find yourself completely unable to let go of self-blame, you may want to seek professional help. Mind you, people do have a go at themselves at times. But unrelenting self-blame is another matter. You can read more about self-acceptance in a broader, deeper sense in Chapter 16.

Anxiety among the rich and famous

So many of our clients seem to think that they're the only people in the world who struggle with anxiety. But we let them know that many millions of people in the UK and in the US, let alone worldwide, suffer from anxiety. Perhaps you won't feel quite so alone if you consider some of the famous people through history who suffered from one or more of the various anxiety disorders discussed in this book.

Elvis Presley, David Bowie, Dennis Bergkamp, Superman (Dean Cain), and Whitney Houston have all been reported to have a fear of flying. Likewise, Albert Einstein and Eleanor Roosevelt are said to have both suffered from fears of social situations. Furthermore, Charles Darwin eventually became a virtual hermit because of his disabling agoraphobia (see Chapter 2), while Robert Frost also battled anxiety.

Billionaire Howard Hughes had many emotional problems, among them, apparently, obsessive-compulsive disorder (see Chapter 2). Hughes insisted on having three copies of a magazine delivered to him. When delivered, Hughes removed the middle magazine with his hands covered in tissue paper. Then he would instruct an assistant to burn the other two magazines. In addition, Hughes had a whole range of other bizarre compulsions involving preparation of his food, the handling of objects, and toileting. OCD received a higher profile following the success of the film *The Aviator*, in which Leonardo DiCaprio plays Howard Hughes.

A very famous figure has spoken of his battle with obsessive compulsive disorder. In an interview in *The Independent* in April 2007, David Beckham admitted that he suffers this problem. He spoke of his addiction to rearranging hotel rooms and lining up cans of soft drinks in his fridge to make 'everything perfect'. Beckham says he has tried to break his cycle of repetitive behaviour but cannot stop.

Finally, a quick search on the Internet shows you that hundreds of celebrities reportedly suffer from all kinds of severe problems with anxiety. Just use a major search engine and type in 'famous people and anxiety'. You'll be surprised by what you find.

Having Second Thoughts About Change

Clearly, no-one likes feeling anxious, tense, and nervous, or having anxiety that may reach such heights that it overwhelms personal resources and the capacity to cope. Chronic, severe anxiety frequently serves as a prelude to serious depression. Obviously, anyone experiencing this torment would jump at the chance to do something about it.

With good intentions, people buy self-help books, attend workshops, and even seek therapy. They fully intend to make meaningful changes in their lives. However, as the old proverb puts it, 'The road to Hell is paved with good intentions.'

Have you ever gone to a health club in January? They're packed with new, enthusiastic members. By mid-March, health clubs return to normal. Like so many New Year's resolutions, the initial burst of resolve too often fades. What happens to all that determination?

When you bought this book, you may have vowed to do something about your anxiety once and for all. Like the January health club enthusiasts, you may still feel motivated and focused. If so, feel free to skip this section.

If you start losing your willpower or your belief in your ability to do something about your anxiety, come back to this section! It can help you get back on track.

What happens to the people at the health clubs in March? Usually, they think that they've simply lost their willpower. Actually, sabotaging thoughts creep into their minds and steal away their motivation. They start to think that they don't have the time or the money, or that they can get into shape later. Such thoughts seduce them into abandoning their goals.

Thoughts about abandoning your quest to overcome anxiety may disrupt your efforts at some point. If so, the first step involves identifying which thought(s) stream through your mind. Then we give you strategies for fighting them off. So now, in the best traditions of the pop chart countdown, our top ten excuses for staying stuck:

10. Anxiety isn't really that big of a problem for me. I thought it was when I bought this book, but my anxiety isn't as bad as for some of the people I've been reading about. Maybe it's not that big a deal.

9. If I try and fail, I'll make a fool out of myself. My friends and family will think I was stupid to even try.

8. Others will think I'm selfish if I try to make things easier and less stressful for myself.

7. I'm afraid of trying and not getting anywhere. That would make me feel even worse than if I did nothing at all. I'd feel like a failure.

6. Feelings can't really be controlled. It's just fooling yourself to think otherwise. You feel the way you feel.

5. I'll do something about my anxiety when I feel the motivation. Right now, I don't really feel like it. I'm sure the motivation will come; I just have to wait for it.

4. Who would I be without my anxiety? That's just who I am. I'm an anxious person; it's just me.

3. I don't believe I can really change. After all, I've been this way my entire life. Books like these don't work anyway.

2. I'm too busy to do anything about my anxiety. These activities look like they take time. I can't fit them into my busy life.

1. The number one reason people stay stuck: I'm too anxious to do anything about my anxiety. It's too overwhelming to tackle. I just don't know if I can handle the additional stress of even thinking about it. Whenever I think about confronting my anxiety, it makes me feel worse.

Look over our preceding list several times. Mull over each excuse and circle any that seem familiar or reasonable to you. Any of these that you agree with will hinder your progress. Now, we have some ways for you to challenge these excuses, no matter how reasonable they may seem.

Deciding Whether You Really Want to Get Going

If any of our top ten excuses for staying stuck resonate with you, then your decision to overcome anxiety is a bit on the wobbly side. Those thoughts can sabotage your best intentions. Don't underestimate their power.

We have three types of strategies for helping you turn your intentions into actions:

✔ **Debate the decision with yourself.** List your excuses for staying stuck and match them with reasons to move ahead.

✔ **Don't wait for a magical motivating moment.** There's no time like the present.

✔ **Kick-start your programme.** Just do it – the sooner, the better!

Half-hearted decisions lead to procrastination and avoiding the task at hand. Anxiety hurts, but though change is hard, do remember that it's pretty tough, and rough, to feel anxious so much of the time. The next section shows you how to push aside the fear of change.

Debating the decision

Pretend that you're judging a debate. One side is arguing for the status quo – in other words, not changing. The other side takes the pro-change position. Ask which side makes the most sense; declare a winner.

Nelson worries about everything. He wakes up early in the morning with thoughts about what he's got to do that day for school. He has nightmares about going to class without his homework and being embarrassed by his teacher. He puts off applying to university for fear that he won't get in, even though his exam results suggest no problems. He feels nervous, tense, and irritable much of the time. Lately, his worries disrupt his concentration to the extent that he daydreams in class. His parents insist that he see a psychologist for help with his anxiety, but Nelson is reluctant, as he doesn't believe that it will help. The counsellor, making up a chart like Table 3-2, helps him debate his unwillingness to work on overcoming his anxiety.

Table 3-2	Nelson's Great Debate
Excuses for Staying Stuck	*Reasons for Moving Forwards*
If I try and fail, I'll make a fool out of myself. My friends and family will think I was stupid to even try.	Quite a few of my friends have seen a psychologist, and I've never thought badly of them, even if one or two of them didn't seem to get much better. At least they tried. Besides, I guess I have a pretty good chance of succeeding; I usually do with most things I work at.
I'm afraid of trying and not getting anywhere. That would make me feel even worse than if I did nothing at all. I'd feel like a failure.	The only real failure would be to not do anything at all. This anxiety keeps me from doing the best I can in school. I run a bigger risk of failing in my studies if I stay stuck.
Feelings can't really be controlled. It's just fooling yourself to think otherwise. You feel the way you feel.	Just because I feel it's hopeless to do anything, doesn't mean it's true. Many people go to therapy for some reason; surely it makes them feel better or the world wouldn't have a zillion therapists.
Who would I be without my anxiety? That's just who I am. I'm an anxious person; it's just me.	Anxiety doesn't define who I am. It just gets in my way. I have many fine qualities that won't change.

Which side wins the debate? We think that the reasons for moving forwards deserve a clear victory.

If you have some excuses for staying stuck, try subjecting them to debate like Nelson did in Table 3-2. List your 'Excuses for Staying Stuck' on the left side of a blank sheet of paper and your 'Reasons for Moving Forwards' on the right. The following questions may help you develop your arguments for moving forwards:

✔ Does my excuse catastrophise? In other words, am I exaggerating the truth?

✔ Can I find any evidence that would contradict my excuse?

✔ Can I think of people to whom my excuse doesn't apply? And if it doesn't apply to them, why should it to me?

✔ Am I trying to predict the future with negative thinking when no-one can ever know the future?

Off to a flying start

Some excuses for staying stuck sap your motivation and will to change. One of our top ten excuses for staying stuck, number 5, hits this issue head on: 'I'll do something about my anxiety when I feel motivated. Right now, I don't really feel like it. I'm sure the motivation will come; I just have to wait for it.'

This excuse is based on a common misconception. Most people think that they need to wait until motivation hits them before acting. Unfortunately, if you operate on that assumption, you may be in for a long wait. That's because facing your fears doesn't particularly feel good. It can even increase your anxiety for a little while. You may never *feel* like tackling it. However, if you start to take action and achieve just a little progress, your motivation surges.

Ellen can't face driving on motorways. She spends an extra hour each day getting to work and back, because she takes the side roads. She really can't afford the time or the extra petrol and the wear and tear to her car.

Ellen decides to get over her fear once and for all. However, each day when she gets into her car, the very thought of trying to drive even a short distance on the motorway makes her anxious, and she loses her resolve. So she rationalises that she'll do something about her problem when the journey gets so bad that she feels sufficiently motivated to deal with her fear.

Many months pass, the journey remains the same, and so does Ellen's fear of driving on motorways. She realises that she may never *want* to confront her phobia. So she decides to force herself to drive on the motorways for just a short distance, whether she feels like it or not. Ellen decides to just drive between two junctions on the motorway near her home on a Sunday. After she gets home, she is surprised to find herself feeling proud of her small accomplishment and actually wants to do more. Each step she takes increases her motivation and her confidence, and she finds this confidence starts to spill over into other areas of her life.

Action generally precedes motivation; if you wait until you feel like overcoming your anxiety, you may wait a lifetime.

Taking baby steps

If you find that the idea of dealing with your anxiety is just too much to handle, you may be struggling with the number 1 excuse for staying stuck: 'I'm too anxious to do anything about my anxiety. It's too overwhelming to tackle. I just don't know if I can handle the additional stress of even thinking about it. Whenever I think about confronting my anxiety, it makes me feel worse.' If so, putting one foot in front of the other may help; take baby steps.

Stop dwelling on the entire task. For example, if you think about all the steps that you'll take over the next five years, that's an incredible amount of walking. Hundreds, if not thousands, of miles await you. The mere thought of all those miles may stress you out.

You may, like many people, wake up early in the morning on some days with a huge list of tasks that you need to complete in the coming week. Ugh. A sense of defeat sets in and you feel like staying in bed for the rest of the day. Dread replaces enthusiasm. If, instead, you clear your mind of the entire agenda and concentrate on only the first item on the list, your distress is likely to diminish, at least a little.

Persevering through the peaks and valleys

A group of psychologists conducted extensive research on how people make important changes, such as quitting smoking, losing weight, and overcoming emotional difficulties. They found that change isn't a straightforward process. It includes a number of stages.

Precontemplation: In this stage, people haven't even given a thought to doing anything about their problems. They may deny having any difficulty at all. If you're reading this book, you're probably not in this stage.

Contemplation: People start thinking about tackling their problems. But at this stage, people feel that taking action is a little out of their reach.

Preparation: In preparation, people develop a plan for change. They gather their resources and make resolutions.

Action: The real work begins, and the plan is put into action.

Maintenance: Now is the time to hold one's ground. People must hang on in there to prevent slipping back.

Termination: The change has become habit; so much so that relapse is less likely, and further work isn't particularly necessary.

These stages look like a straight line from precontemplation to termination, but what the psychologists found is that people bounce around the stages in various ways. They may go from contemplation to action without having made adequate preparation. Others may reach the maintenance stage and give up on their efforts, slipping back to the precontemplation stage.

Many successful changers bounce back and forth through these stages a number of times before finally achieving their goals. So don't get discouraged if that happens to you. Keep your goal in mind and reinitiate your efforts if you slip. If at first you don't succeed – yep – try, try, and try again.

Paula, for example, is about to put this strategy into play. Paula has social phobia. She can't stand the idea of attending social functions. She feels that the moment that she walks into a group, all eyes focus on her, which sends her anxiety through the roof. She desperately wants to change. But the idea of attending large parties or work social events overwhelms her with terror. Look at Table 3-3 to see how Paula broke the task down into baby steps.

Table 3-3	Paula's Baby Steps to Success
Goals	*Step-by-step Breakdown of Actions*
Ultimate goal	Going to a large party, staying the entire time, and talking with numerous people without fear.
Intermediate goal	Attending a small party, staying a little while, and talking to a couple of people although feeling a little scared.
Small goal	Going to a work-related social event, staying 30 minutes, talking to at least one other person in spite of some anxiety.
First baby step	Phoning a friend and asking her to go to lunch in spite of anxiety.

This simple strategy works, because the overwhelming task is broken down into manageable pieces. Sit down and chart your ultimate goal, and then chart a goal that isn't quite so lofty that can serve as a stepping stone and an intermediate goal. Then work out the action that would be required of you to meet a small goal. If your intermediate goal feels doable, you can start with it. If not, break it down further. It doesn't matter how small you make your first step. Anything that moves you just a little in the right direction can get you going and increase your confidence one step at a time.

Considering the cons and pros

You may think that it's selfish to reduce the demands others are making of you, which have led to you feeling overwhelmed and anxious. But the truth is that meeting all their demands and sacrificing your own wants and needs may well not be the answer. Unless you make space so you can fill your own needs, you quite possibly will become anxious and stressed. Then your anxiety may well make you unhappy, angry, and even physically unwell – and then what sort of condition will you be in to support others? So looking after yourself no longer becomes selfish, but can be seen as a way of helping you be in the right space to help others.

Another possibility is that maybe you suffer from anxiety, but when it comes to doing something about it, you start thinking that yours isn't all that bad after all. If so, you may be *rationalising* and letting excuse number 10 get in the way: 'Anxiety isn't really that big of a problem for me. I thought it was when I bought this book, but my anxiety isn't as bad as for some of the people I've been reading about. Maybe it's not that big a deal.'

On the other hand, perhaps your anxiety doesn't warrant doing anything about it. If so, then that's wonderful! Give this book to a friend who needs it more than you do! But how can you figure out whether you're in denial? Pondering the pros and cons of conquering your anxiety can help you.

Mike is in charge of the accounts department of a large manufacturing plant. He has huge responsibilities, multiple deadlines, and difficult people to supervise. He depends on many people to submit figures for his quarterly report, but sometimes they fail to deliver on time, and Mike needs to confront them. Unfortunately, Mike dreads conflict and avoids reminding them. The stress of waiting makes Mike feel nauseous, tense, and irritable. He knows that he has anxiety, but he reckons that he's managed so far and therefore questions whether it's worth trying to change.

Mike ponders the pros and cons of tackling his problem. Putting his concerns in perspective, he organises his thoughts for taking action versus his fears on paper. (Look at Table 3-4 in this chapter to see how Mike mapped out his pros and cons.) Mike starts by listing the cons of taking action, because he's more fully aware of what those are.

Table 3-4	Mike's Cons and Pros for Taking Action
Cons of Taking Action	**Pros of Taking Action**
It will make me more anxious to confront people.	I suffer from anxiety anyway. I worry that I'll get in trouble if I can't get these people to produce their figures on time. If I confront the people who I need to, maybe they'll be more co-operative.
People may not like me if I confront them.	I avoid people so much that they don't even know who I am. So what if a few people don't like me? Feeling less worried about people liking me sounds pretty good.
I'm happy in my job most of the time. My quarterly report just happens once a quarter.	Yes, it only happens once a quarter, but I dread the quarterly report for weeks in advance. Getting rid of the dread sounds worth doing.

When Mike considers his cons and pros carefully, he makes the decision to do something about his discomfort. You can use Mike's chart in Table 3-4 as an example to help you chart your reasons for and against taking action. If your motivation starts fading because you're not sure how serious your problem is, take the time to reflect thoroughly. Generate as many reasons as you can.

Chapter 4

Watching Worries Ebb and Flow

Anxiety may feel like it will never go away. Believing that you have no control over it and that stress invades your every waking moment is easy. This chapter helps you to realise that anxiety actually has an ebb and flow. Then we show you how taking a few minutes to write down your feelings each day may discharge a little of your anxiety and possibly improve your health. Finally, we help you understand that progress too, like anxiety, ebbs and flows.

Following Your Fears All the Way Down the Line

One of the best early steps that you can take to conquer anxiety is to simply chart it every day in a couple of different ways. Why would you want to do that? After all, you're fully aware that you're anxious. Well, watching your worries actually starts the process of change. You discover important patterns, triggers, and insights into your anxiety.

Observing your anxiety from head to toe

Observing anxiety fulfils several useful functions. First, monitoring forces you to be aware of your emotions. Avoiding and running away from troubling emotions only causes them to escalate. Secondly, you'll see that your anxiety goes up and down throughout the day, which is not quite as upsetting as thinking it rules every moment of your life. And you're likely to discover that recording your anxiety levels can help you take charge and feel more in control of what's going on inside you. Finally, keeping track helps you see how you're progressing in your efforts to deal with your distress. Vanessa's story shows you how.

Vanessa complains to her friends that she's the most nervous person on the planet and that she's close to a nervous breakdown. Recently, her father had heart surgery and her husband lost his job. Vanessa feels completely out of control and says that her anxiety never stops. When her therapist suggests that she start tracking her anxiety, she tells him, 'You've got to be kidding. I don't need to do that. I can tell you right now that I'm anxious all the time. There's no let up.' He urges her to go ahead and try anyway.

Table 4-1 shows what Vanessa comes up with in her first week of rating and recording her anxiety. On a scale from 1 (complete calm) to 10 (total panic), Vanessa rates the level of anxiety that she experiences at around the same time in the morning, then again in the afternoon, and later in the evening.

Table 4-1	Vanessa's Day-by-day Anxiety Levels			
Day	**Morning**	**Afternoon**	**Evening**	**Daily Average**
Sunday	4	6	8	6
Monday	6	7	9	7.3
Tuesday	5	6	6	5.7
Wednesday	4	5	7	5.3
Thursday	3	8	8	6.3
Friday	5	9	9	7.7
Saturday	3	5	5	4.3
Average	**4.3**	**6.6**	**7.4**	**6.1**

Vanessa discovers a few things. First, she notices that her anxiety is routinely less intense in the morning. It also tends to escalate in the afternoon and peak in the evenings. With only one week's records, she can't discern whether her anxiety level is decreasing, increasing, or remaining stable. However, she notices that she is feeling a little better simply because she feels like she's starting to take charge of her problem. She also realises that some days are better than others and that her anxiety varies rather than overwhelming her all the time.

Boosting booster shots

Research into the value of expressing emotions in diaries spans a wide range of populations and problems. One of the more interesting studies looked at healthy medical students who had not yet had their required hepatitis B vaccinations. The researchers speculated that writing about traumatic events may result in improved immunity. Hepatitis B vaccinations come in a series of three shots. Prior to receiving the first shot, one group of students was assigned by researchers to write about past traumatic events daily for four days. The other group wrote about non-personal issues. At four months and even after six months following the shots, the blood of the students in the traumatic writing group had more antibodies against the hepatitis B virus than did the blood of those in the other group.

Record your anxiety in a notebook for a few weeks. Carry your anxiety-tracking notebook with you and try to fill it out at the same times each day. Notice patterns or differences in intensity.

Writing about your worries – warts and all

Millions of people keep a diary or journal at some point in their lives. Some develop daily writing as a lifelong habit. Logically, people who keep diaries must feel that they get something out of their writing or they wouldn't do it.

Keeping a diary of life's emotionally significant events has surprising benefits:

- ✔ Diary writing appears to decrease the number of visits people make to the doctor for physical complaints.
- ✔ Writing increases the production of T cells, which are beneficial to the immune system.
- ✔ Keeping a diary about emotional events improved the exam results of a group of college students compared with the results of those who wrote about trivial matters.
- ✔ Unemployed workers who wrote about the trauma of losing their jobs found new employment more quickly than those who did not.

Throwing out the rule book

Diary writing doesn't have rules. You can write about anything, anywhere, and at any time. However, if you want the full benefits of writing in a diary, we encourage you to write about feelings and the emotionally important events in your life. Write about anything that troubles you during the day and/or past difficulties. Spend a little time on it.

Writing about past traumas may bring considerable relief. However, if you find that the task floods you with overwhelming grief or anxiety, you'll probably find it helpful to seek professional assistance.

Counting your blessings: An antidote for anxiety

Writing about your distressing feelings makes a great start. However, if you'd like to make a greater impact, take a few extra minutes and write about what you feel grateful for each day. Why? Because positive emotions help counter-act negative emotions. Writing about your advantages and blessings improves mood, increases optimism, and may benefit your health.

At first glance, you may think that you have little to be grateful for. Anxiety can so easily cloud vision. Did your mother ever urge you to finish everything on your plate because of the 'starving children in Africa?' As much as we think that pushing children to eat is a bad idea, her notion to consider those less fortunate has value. Take some time to ponder the positive events and people in your life.

- ✔ **Kindnesses:** Think about those who have extended kindness to you.

- ✔ **Education:** Obviously, you can read; that's a blessing for you compared with the millions in the world with no chance for an education.

- ✔ **Nourishment:** You probably aren't starving to death, while, as your mother may have noted, millions are.

- ✔ **Home:** Do you live in a cardboard box or do you have a roof over your head?

- ✔ **Pleasure:** Can you smell flowers, hear birds sing, or touch the soft fur of a pet?

Sources of possible gratitude abound – freedom, health, companionship, and so on. Everyone has a different list. You can find yours by following Caroline's example.

Caroline, a single mother, worries about money, managing her house, and especially about her children: Tom, aged 15, and Julia, 12. She worries about the effect that her divorce had on her kids and tries to be mother and father as well as teacher and police officer to them. Sometimes, she just feels like crying. When the headmaster calls to tell her that a teacher has caught her son smoking cannabis in the school grounds, she falls apart. The court orders counselling for the entire family. The therapist suggests keeping a diary of hassles and blessings for both Caroline and her son Tom. Look at Caroline's first entries in Table 4-2 in this chapter.

Table 4-2	Caroline's Daily Hassles and Gratitude Diary	
Time of Day	*Hassles*	*Blessings*
Morning	As usual, I had to wake Tom three or four times even though his alarm went off. He barely talked to me at breakfast and was almost late for school. I worry so much that he'll fail everything. What would I do then? I want so much for him to be happy in life.	I can at least appreciate the fact that my kids are healthy. We have a nice home, and although I feel money is tight sometimes, no-one is starving here.
Afternoon	At work, I have been put in charge of the new Blare account. I don't know if I can handle this much responsibility. It makes me nervous just thinking about organising all the people involved.	Wait a second, I have a great job and a new promotion. The boss must think that I'm good at my work even if I worry about it.
Evening	Dinner was the usual frozen stir-fry. Tom didn't come home from football training until everything was cold. Julia watched TV and said little.	I'm grateful for the fact that Tom is interested in football. It will help keep him away from the wrong crowd. Julia is the sweetest kid there ever was, even though she watches too much TV.

Certainly, Caroline needs to work with her son about the incident at school and a few other issues. But when her anxiety rises to extremes, she can't be the parent she wants to be.

Keeping a diary helps Caroline put a different perspective on her problems. She realises that she's been so uptight about her kids that she hasn't taken the time to notice the good things about them and about her own life. Like most people, Caroline has her share of hassles and blessings. Writing about her hassles discharges a little of the emotion that she has bottled up. Writing about what she feels grateful for helps to counteract some of her negative thoughts.

Consider keeping a diary as Caroline did. You can use Table 4-2 as a format for your own daily notes. Even if you don't think that it can help you, try it for a few days. You may be surprised.

The power of positive psychology

The field of psychology focused on negative emotions for most of the 20th century. Psychologists studied depression, anxiety, schizophrenia, behaviour disorders, and a whole host of other maladies. Only recently has the field looked at the pluses of positive emotions, the characteristics of happy people, and the components of wellbeing. People who feel grateful usually say that they feel happier as well.

One study assigned people to three groups. The first group wrote only about the hassles of everyday life. The researchers asked the second group to write about emotionally neutral events. The third group recorded experiences that they were grateful for. All the groups performed this task merely once a week for ten weeks. At the end of the experiment (reported in full in Volume 19, 2000, of the *Journal of Social and Clinical Psychology*), the group that wrote about gratitude exercised more, had fewer physical complaints, and felt more optimistic than those in the other two groups. That such an easy, simple task can be so beneficial is surprising.

Consider giving thanks and appreciating life's gifts from small to large.

Sizing Up Success

You may feel some benefit from simply rating your anxiety on a daily basis and from your diary, but don't expect large improvements overnight. Change takes time. Sometimes it takes a number of weeks before a positive direction emerges. After all, you spent much of your life feeling anxious; give change time as well.

You should also know that improvement does not happen in a constant, smooth fashion. Rather, it takes a jagged, mountainous course with many ups and downs. You'll have peaks – times when you feel that you're on top of the world and on the verge of conquering your anxiety. But you'll also slip into valleys, even down cliffs, and you may feel as though you're on the edge of failure and despair.

Realise that if you're standing in the middle of one of the valleys, it looks like a long climb. You may even feel like you're making no progress at all, because all that you see are peaks around you. These are not the times for evaluating your progress. However, the advantage of a valley is that it can tell you much about what trips you up. So if you're in a valley, rather than catastrophise, take the opportunity to reflect on the elements that may have led you there, and know that things will get better.

If you don't start feeling better after a number of weeks, or if you start feeling utterly hopeless, you should consider seeking professional advice.

Part II
Understanding Thought Remedies

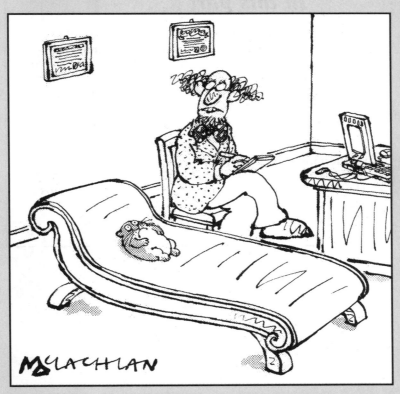

'I wouldn't let fear of water
bother you too much, Mr Lemming.'

In this part . . .

We talk about one of the most effective therapies for anxiety and show you methods for tracking your anxiety-arousing thoughts along with ways to change anxious thoughts into calmer thinking. Next, we describe the anxiety-provoking assumptions that underlie many anxious thoughts. You can discover which anxiety-provoking assumptions plague you and how you can do something about them.

Furthermore, you'll see that the very words you use to think about yourself and the world can intensify anxiety. The good news is that you can replace your worry words with more reasonable language. In so doing, you reduce your anxiety.

Chapter 5

Becoming a Thought Detective

*U*nderstanding anxiety doesn't make you immune to experiencing it! One of the authors of this book, Elaine, was in Hong Kong a few years ago. She writes, 'The conference was over, the presentation had been successful, and now was my time. I decided on a picnic at the top of Victoria Hill. Sauntering along the road, I saw a sign pointing through the woods, showing the walk around the top, and the way back to the train. A farther sign pointed the road route – half the time, but not nearly so enticing. No contest.

I was about half way along, thinking how blessed I was – all alone on this wonderful wooded walk, with only birds for company, so peaceful, so away from it all – when I suddenly thought, "And no-one knows I'm here!" Such freedom. And then as if a switch was thrown, in crept those thoughts – I'm all alone. No-one knows I'm here. What if I meet an unpleasant fate? They'll never find me. A colleague told me a crew member had disappeared without trace in Hong Kong. Disappeared without trace in Hong Kong. No-one knows I'm here – they'll never find me.

I quickened my pace, almost running, but became aware of tree roots on the path. If I trip, fall down the side, break a bone – no-one will ever find me. . . (Yes, they will, eventually, by the smell!) Having thoroughly terrified myself, I certainly was in no mood to stop for my picnic. And finally reaching the end of the walk and seeing a family group, I've never been so delighted to not have a space all to myself.

Yet the walk and the woods didn't change in any way. Only my perception of them. My perception started the rising feelings of physical anxiety and increasingly catastrophic thoughts which, though I did challenge them, did not fully subside until I left the situation, which had changed from peace, tranquillity and beauty to terrifying isolation, where even the trees began to seem menacing.'

In this chapter, we show you how powerfully your thoughts influence your emotions and perceptions. You can become a thought detective, able to uncover the thoughts that contribute to anxious feelings. We show you how to gather evidence and put your thoughts on trial. You can see how thoughts all too easily trigger your anxiety, and we give you proven techniques for transforming your anxious thoughts into calm thoughts.

Distinguishing Thoughts from Feelings

Psychologists often ask questions of their clients to find out how they feel about recent events in their lives. Frequently, clients answer with how they *think* about the events rather than how they *feel*. For example, Dr Wolfe had a highly anxious client named Jim, who complained about his marriage in the following manner:

> **Dr Wolfe:** How did you feel when your wife said you were irresponsible?
>
> **Jim:** I thought she was really out of line.
>
> **Dr Wolfe:** I see. But how did you *feel* about what she said?
>
> **Jim:** She's at least as irresponsible as I am.
>
> **Dr Wolfe:** I suppose that's possible. But again, what were your *feelings*, your emotional reaction to what she said? Were you anxious, even angry or upset?
>
> **Jim:** Well, I couldn't believe she could accuse me of that.
>
> **Dr Wolfe:** I wonder if we should take some time to help you get in touch with your feelings?

Perhaps Jim is extremely anxious and worried that his wife will leave him, or possibly he's angry with her. Maybe her stinging criticism hurt him. Both Jim and Dr Wolfe could learn a great deal from knowing more about what Jim is feeling, rather than only the thoughts he has when he gets upset.

This example shows that people may not always know how to describe what they're feeling. If you don't always know what you're feeling, that's okay.

Beating the blues

People often have trouble identifying and labelling their feelings and emotions, especially negative ones. Actually, the difficulty makes sense for two reasons.

First, emotions often hurt. No-one wants to feel sadness, grief, anxiety, or fear. One simple solution is to *avoid* feelings entirely, and many creative ways to avoid emotions are available. Unfortunately, most of these methods can be destructive.

- **Alcohol and drug abuse:** When people feel bad, numbing their emotions with drugs and alcohol provides a temporary, artificial emotional lift; of course, habitually doing so can lead to addiction, ill health, and sometimes even death.

- **Alternative activities:** Athletics, entertainment, hobbies, television, surfing the Internet, and many other activities can be employed, but only after you have identified and dealt with the bad feelings. Unlike the other preceding strategies, alternative activities are a good thing. It's only when you try to distract yourself and don't deal with the feelings, trying to cover up or avoid them, that alternative activities turn into distraction, which can become problematic.

- **Denial and repression:** One strategy for not feeling is to fool yourself and pretend that nothing is wrong.

- **Comfort eating:** Heading for the fridge or the food cupboard when you are feeling anxious but not actually hungry, and then concentrating on the sensations of eating and drinking, can be another way of paying less attention to what you are feeling. Certain foods, in particular chocolate, can actually make you feel better in the short term. But if you then start gaining weight, this can make you more anxious and more prone to comfort eating. You can become caught in a vicious cycle.

- **Sensation seeking:** High-risk activities, such as sexual promiscuity and compulsive gambling, can push away distress for a while.

- **Workaholism:** Some people work all the time rather than think about what's disturbing them.

The second reason that identifying, expressing, and labelling feelings is such a struggle for people is because they're taught from an early age that they shouldn't feel certain feelings. Parents, teachers, friends, and relatives bombard kids with 'don't feel' messages. Look at these examples of 'don't feel' messages that you've probably heard before:

- Big boys don't cry.
- Don't be a baby.

- ✔ Don't be a chicken.
- ✔ Don't be a scaredy-cat.
- ✔ Don't be so ridiculous.
- ✔ Get over it!
- ✔ Grow up.
- ✔ It couldn't possibly hurt that badly.
- ✔ Pull yourself together.
- ✔ Stop crying or I'll give you something to cry about!

That many people are described as being out of touch with their feelings is no wonder. The problem with the habitual tendency to avoid feelings is that you don't find out how to cope with or resolve the underlying issues. Chronic avoidance creates a certain kind of low-level stress that builds over time.

Getting in touch with your feelings

Noticing your emotions can help you gain insight and discover how to cope more effectively. If you don't know what your feelings are, when they occur, or what brings them on, you can't do much about changing them.

We realise that some people are aware of their feelings and know all too well when they're feeling the slightest amount of anxiety or worry. If you're one of those, feel free to skip or skim the rest of this section.

Take some time right now to assess your mood. First, notice your breathing. Is it rapid and shallow or slow and deep? Notice your posture. Are you relaxed or is some part of your body in an uncomfortable position? Check out all your physical sensations. Look for sensations of tension, queasiness, tightness, dizziness, or heaviness. No matter what you find, just study it and sit with the sensations for a while. Then you may ask yourself what *feeling* captures the essence of those sensations. Of course, at this moment you may not have any strong feelings. If so, your breathing is rhythmic and your posture relaxed. Even if that's the case, notice what it feels like to be calm. At other times, notice your stronger sensations.

Feeling words describe your physical and mental reactions to events.

Perhaps we're presuming too much, but because you're reading this book, we guess that you or someone close to you wants to know about anxiety. So we've given you the following vocabulary list for describing anxious feelings. The next time you can't find the right words to describe how you feel, one of the words that follows may get you started.

Denial ain't just a river in Egypt

In *Gone With the Wind*, Scarlett O'Hara says time and again, 'I'll think about that tomorrow. After all, tomorrow is another day.' What a nice, easy solution to tough times – just push the issue out of the way. But we're discovering more about the costs of avoiding and repressing emotions. According to researchers at Adelphi University and the University of Michigan, people who declare themselves as mentally healthy over the years when other evidence shows they're not have higher heart rates and blood pressure in response to stress than people who own up to their emotional difficulties or those who truly don't have problems at the time. Studies also show that when people write about their emotions on a daily basis, their immune systems improve, even if a person is suffering from AIDS. Amazing stuff. Check out Chapter 4 for more on keeping a diary.

Afraid	Panicked
Anxious	Petrified
Agitated	Self-conscious
Apprehensive	Shaky
Disturbed	Tense
Fearful	Terrified
Frightened	Timid
Insecure	Uneasy
Nervous	Uptight
Obsessed	Worried

We're sure that we've missed a few dozen possibilities on the word list, and maybe you have a favourite way to describe your anxiety. That's fine. What we encourage you to do is to start paying attention to your feelings and bodily sensations. You may want to look over this list a number of times and ask whether you've felt any of these emotions recently. Try not to make judgements about your feelings. They may be trying to tell you something useful.

Anxiety and fear also have a positive function: they ready your mind and body for danger. Bad feelings only cause problems when you feel bad repeatedly over a long period of time in the absence of a clear threat.

Negative emotions have an adaptive role to play. They alert you to danger and prepare you to respond. For example, if King Kong knocks on your door, adrenaline floods your body and mobilises you to fight him or run like hell!

That's good for situations like that. But if you feel like King Kong is knocking on your door on a regular basis, and he's not even in the area, your anxious feelings cause you more harm than good.

Whether King Kong is knocking at your door or not, identifying anxious, fearful, or worried feelings can help you deal with them far more effectively than if you avoid them. When you can see what's going on, you can focus on what to do about your predicament more easily than you can sitting in the dark.

Getting in touch with your thoughts

Just as some people don't have much idea about what they're feeling, others have trouble knowing what they're thinking when they're anxious, worried, or stressed. Because thoughts have a powerful influence on feelings, psychologists like to ask their clients what they were thinking when they started to feel upset. Sometimes clients describe feelings rather than thoughts. For example, Dr Baker had the following dialogue with Susan, a client who has severe anxiety:

Dr Baker: So when your supervisor told you off, you said you felt panicked. What thoughts went through your mind?

Susan: Well, I just felt horrible. I couldn't stand it.

Dr Baker: I know; it must have felt really awful. But I'm curious about what thoughts went through your mind. What did you say to yourself about your supervisor's comments?

Susan: I felt my heart pounding in my chest. I don't think I really had any thoughts actually.

Dr Baker: That's possible. Sometimes our thoughts escape us for a while. But I wonder, if you think about it now, what did those comments mean to you? What did you think would happen?

Susan: I'm shaking right now just thinking about it.

As this example illustrates, people don't always know what's going on in their heads when they feel anxious. Sometimes you may not have clear, identifiable thoughts when you feel worried or stressed. That's perfectly normal.

The challenge is to find out what the stressful event *means* to you. That will tell you what your thoughts are. Consider the example you've just read about. Susan may have felt panicked because she feared losing her job, or she may have thought her boss's criticism meant that she was incompetent. The reprimand may have also triggered memories of her abusive father. Knowing what thoughts stand behind the feelings can help both Dr Baker and Susan plan the next step.

Tapping into your triggers

 If you're like Susan, you don't always know what's going on in your mind when you feel anxious. To figure it out, you need to first identify the *situation* that preceded your upset. Focus on what happened moments before your troublesome feelings. Perhaps you

- Opened your mail and found that your credit card debt had skyrocketed
- Heard someone say something that bothered you
- Read a poor end of term report from your child's school
- Are wondering why your partner is so late coming home
- Just got off the scales, having seen a number that you didn't like
- Noticed that your chest feels tight and your heart is racing for no good reason

On the other hand, sometimes your anxiety-triggering event hasn't even happened yet. You may be just sitting around and *wham* – an avalanche of anxiety crashes around you. Other people wake up at 4 a.m. with worries marching through their minds. What's the trigger then? Well, it can be an image or a fear of some future event. See the following examples of anxiety-triggering thoughts and images:

- I'll never have enough money for retirement.
- Did I turn off the cooker before I left the house?
- We'll never meet the publication deadline!
- No-one is going to like my speech tomorrow.
- What if I'm made redundant tomorrow?
- What if my partner leaves me?

Listen as Veronica searches for her anxiety-triggering event:

Veronica works in the university admissions office. The university offers her free tuition for two classes per term. One day, Veronica's manager suggests that she consider taking a course in business administration to increase her chances of getting a promotion in the department. Later, she finds herself feeling unusually anxious. She doesn't know why.

However, after she thinks about it for a while, Veronica realises that the trigger for her anxiety is the thought of studying and having to sit through exams. She has always hated tests. Veronica never considered going to university because she's so anxious about taking tests. Veronica's anxiety trigger is the image of a future event – the idea of taking a test.

Thought-catching

If you know your feelings and the triggers for those feelings, you're ready to become a thought detective. Thoughts powerfully influence emotions. The event may serve as the trigger, but it isn't what directly leads to your anxiety. The meaning that the event holds for you causes the anxiety, and your thoughts reflect that meaning.

For example, suppose your spouse is 45 minutes late coming home from work. You could think *anxious* thoughts:

- Maybe she's had an accident.
- She's probably having an affair.

Or you may have different thoughts that don't cause so much anxiety:

- I love having time alone with the kids.
- I like having time alone to work on house projects.
- The traffic must be really bad tonight.

Some thoughts create anxiety; others feel good; still others don't stir up much feeling at all. Capturing your thoughts and seeing how they trigger anxiety and connect to your feelings is important. If you're not sure what thoughts are in your head when you're anxious, you can do something to find them.

First, focus on the anxiety trigger. Think about it for a while; don't rush it. Then ask yourself some questions about the trigger. The following list of what we call *minding-your-mind questions* can help you identify your thoughts or the meaning that the event holds for you:

- Specifically, what about this event do I find upsetting?
- What's the worst that could happen?
- How may this event affect my life?
- How may this event affect the way others see me?
- Does this remind me of anything in my past that bothered me?
- What would my parents say about this event?
- How may this event affect the way I see myself?

Veronica (you remember her name from earlier in this chapter) suffers from test anxiety. Look at her answers to a few of the following questions from the minding-your-mind list. Her answers indicate what thoughts she has about exams.

> ✔ **What's the worst that could happen?**
>
> I could fail the test and my boss would find out.
>
> ✔ **How may this event affect the way others see me?**
>
> My boss and my colleagues will know how stupid I am.
>
> ✔ **How may this event affect the way I see myself?**
>
> I'll finally know for sure that I'm the loser I've always thought I may be.

Even though earlier, Veronica couldn't explain why tests made her so anxious, answering these questions brings her hidden thoughts about exams to light. No wonder she feels so anxious. Perhaps you'll discover some hidden thoughts of your own if you ask yourself these questions about your anxiety triggers.

Here's Andrew's story:

Andrew loves his work. He designs computer systems for a living and relishes creating complex systems to meet his clients' needs. The management appreciates Andrew's expertise and rewards him with a promotion and the opportunity to design a major system for a national laboratory. Andrew can't wait to begin, at least until he realises that part of the project involves giving a number of talks to groups of managers and scientists. Andrew's heart races and he perspires profusely at the mere thought of speaking in front of a group. Andrew has been terrified of speaking in front of an audience since junior school, but he has no idea why.

Andrew has a rather common fear – the fear of speaking in public. He answers a few of the minding-your-mind questions:

> ✔ **Specifically, what about this event do I find upsetting?**
>
> I'll look silly and forget what I wanted to say.
>
> ✔ **How may this event affect my life?**
>
> They'll think I'm incapable of putting this system together, and I'll lose the sale.
>
> ✔ **How may this event affect the way others see me?**
>
> They'll know how scared I am and think I'm a fool. Those scientists know more than I do.

When you work with the minding-your-mind questions, use your imagination. Brainstorm and take your time. Even though our examples don't answer all the questions, you may find it useful to build on these ideas.

Tracking Your Thoughts, Triggers, and Feelings

Monitoring your thoughts, feelings, and whatever triggers your anxiety paves the way for change. This simple strategy helps you focus on your personal pattern of stress and worry. The very act of paying attention brings your thinking process to light. This clarification helps you gain a new perspective.

If recording your thoughts, feelings, and triggers makes you more anxious, that's okay. It's common. Many other techniques in this book should help you deal with any additional anxiety, especially the ones in this chapter for challenging your thoughts. But if the techniques in this book don't help you, consider seeking professional help.

Try using the thought-therapy Chart in Table 5-1 to connect your thoughts, feelings, and anxiety triggers. To show you how to use the chart, we've filled it in with Veronica's notes. When you monitor the triggers, include the day, time, place, people involved, and what was going on. When you record your anxious thoughts, use the minding-your-mind questions in the 'Thought-catching' section earlier in this chapter. Finally, write down your anxious feelings and physical sensations, and rate the severity of those feelings. Use 1 to represent almost no anxiety at all and 100 to indicate the most severe anxiety imaginable. (Sort of like how you may feel if 100 snakes suddenly appeared slithering around your bedroom!)

Table 5-1	Thought-Therapy Chart		
Circumstances of Trigger	*Anxious Thoughts*	*Feelings and Sensations*	*Rating*
Tuesday morning	If I take this training course, I'll fail, and my boss will find out.	Anxious	70
At work	I'll never get ahead in this job.	Queasy stomach	60
My boss suggested that I take the training.	I'm really stupid.	Tension	65

You can use this simple technique to monitor your anxious feelings, thoughts, and triggers. Simply design your own thought-therapy chart using the headings of Table 5-1. Keep track of your thoughts and feelings and what triggers them, and look for patterns.

Ray discovers that he feels anxious on most Mondays. He realises that he tends to sleep late on Sunday morning and therefore has trouble falling asleep on Sunday night. A lack of sleep usually makes him more susceptible to anxiety triggers. What doesn't bother him on Tuesday, stresses him out on Monday. Ray changes his sleep habits and feels a little less anxious on Mondays.

Marion, a primary school teacher, tracks her triggers, thoughts, and feelings for a month. She isn't surprised to discover that she feels anxious about the possibility of receiving criticism. She notices herself shaking the day that the headmistress observes her class for her annual assessment. She finds it difficult to nail down her thoughts at first, so she uses the minding-your-mind questions in the 'Thought-catching' section earlier in this chapter. She asks the question, 'What would your parents say about this?' Marion actually hears her mother's caustic voice in her head saying, 'You'll never amount to anything if you can't even look after your own room.'

Marion realises how critical her mother was and how much her mother's harshness hurt her. Just figuring that out helps Marion see that she is expecting the headmistress to be like her mother. When she thinks about it, she remembers the headmistress giving her a number of compliments about her teaching. She understands that a negative evaluation is unlikely. This insight alone reduces her anxiety.

Although monitoring may produce useful insights that reduce your anxiety a bit, you, like most people, may need a little more assistance. The next section shows you how to tackle your anxious thoughts and make them manageable.

Tackling Your Thoughts: Thought Therapy

We have three simple strategies for tackling your anxious thoughts:

- ✔ **Thought court:** Take your thoughts to court and sift through the evidence.

- ✔ **Rethink risk:** Recalculate the odds of your anxious thoughts coming true – most people overestimate the odds.

- ✔ **Worst-case scenarios:** Re-examine your ability to cope even if the worst does occur. Most people underestimate their coping resources.

We met Veronica in the section 'Tapping into your triggers', earlier in this chapter. She tracks her anxious thoughts about sitting exams. But she never questions them. She remains anxious and convinced that if she undertakes the course, she will surely fail. And everyone will realise how stupid she is. Veronica needs more than monitoring to deal with her anxious thoughts. She must go to thought court to review the evidence for and against her habitual way of thinking.

Weighing the evidence: Anxiety on trial

The thoughts that lead to your anxious feelings have most likely been around a long time. Most people consider their thoughts to be true. They don't question them. You may be surprised to discover that many of your thoughts don't hold up under scrutiny. If you carefully gather and weigh the evidence, you just may find that your thoughts rest on a foundation made of sand.

Keep in mind that gathering evidence to challenge your thoughts when you're feeling really anxious isn't always easy to do. At those times, it's hard to consider that your thoughts may be inaccurate. When that's the case, you'll be better off waiting until you calm down before hunting for the evidence. At other times, if your anxiety isn't too out of control, you may be able to find evidence. You may find it useful to consider the following *evidence-gathering questions* when judging the accuracy of your anxious thoughts.

✔ Have I had thoughts like these at other times in my life? Have my dire predictions ever come true?

✔ Do I have experiences that would contradict my thoughts in any way?

✔ Is this situation really as awful as I'm making it out to be?

✔ A year from now, how much concern will I have with this issue?

✔ Am I thinking this will happen just because I'm feeling anxious and worried? Am I basing my conclusion mostly on my feelings or on the true evidence?

Feelings are always valid in the sense that you feel what you feel. But they are not evidence for supporting anxious predictions. For example, if you feel extremely anxious about taking an exam, the anxiety is not evidence of how you will perform.

These evidence-gathering questions can help you discover evidence for and against your anxious or worrisome thoughts. Take a look at Veronica's notes again in Table 5-1, earlier in this chapter, and her collection of evidence that follows in Table 5-2. Veronica used the evidence-gathering questions in this section and then created a table to list the evidence against her anxious predictions in the second column of the table.

Table 5-2	Weighing the Evidence
Evidence Supporting My Anxious Thoughts	*Evidence Against My Anxious Thoughts*
I know that my boss will find out if I don't pass, because the university pays for my tuition.	There's no evidence that my boss will find out if I don't pass. However, even if she does, she'll probably just feel sympathy for me.
I almost failed chemistry in my final year of school.	At school, chemistry was the only subject that gave me trouble. I managed pretty well with all the others.
My father always said that I was slow to learn.	The reason that I feel stupid is probably because of my father; no-one else ever said that. Besides, feelings aren't really evidence!
I don't feel bright.	My boss wouldn't have suggested that I take this course unless she thought I could do it. Besides, feelings are not evidence.
My best friend got better exam results than I did, and she's at university now. I must be an idiot.	My best friend was just more confident than me; that's why she's at university. My results were good enough.
I've been in this job for two years and haven't yet been promoted.	Nobody gets promoted here unless they take these courses. Logically, that's the only reason I haven't been promoted.

After completing the task, Veronica makes a new judgement about her anxious thoughts. Veronica realises that the evidence supporting her anxious thoughts doesn't hold up to scrutiny. Upon reflection, she sees that many of her feelings of inferiority stem from a critical father. Furthermore, she's surprised by how much evidence actually supports an alternative view – that she's actually quite capable. Thus she has a change of heart and, more importantly, her anxiety decreases. She decides to take the course and do the best she can.

Consider filling out your own chart so that you can weigh the evidence carefully. Use the same column headings and format as in Table 5-2. Be creative and come up with as much evidence for and against your anxious thoughts as you can.

Don't forget to use the evidence-gathering questions listed earlier in this section if you need help generating ideas.

Decide whether you truly think that your anxious thoughts hold water. If they don't, you just may start taking them less seriously, and your anxiety rating could drop a point or two.

Although recording your anxious thoughts and weighing the evidence just once may prove to be helpful, practice really can make perfect. The longer you keep at it, and the more times you record your anxious thoughts, balancing them against the real evidence, the more you'll gain. Many of our clients find that thought records kept regularly for three or four months alleviate a considerable number of their negative feelings.

⚘ *Rethinking risk*

Another important way to challenge your anxious thoughts is to look at how you assess probabilities. When you feel anxious, like many people, you may *overestimate the odds* of unwanted events actually occurring. It's easy to do. For example, when's the last time you heard a news bulletin reporting that no-one got bitten by a snake today, or that half a million planes took off and landed today and not a single one crashed? No wonder people overestimate disaster. Because dramatic events grab our attention, we focus on these events rather than routine ones. That's why it's useful to think about the real, objective odds of your predicted catastrophe happening.

Thoughts are just thoughts. Subject them to a reality test.

Mary from Manchester fears flying. Her father-in-law, who lived in Italy, dies unexpectedly. Mary drives across Europe to the funeral rather than join her husband who chooses to fly. Not only is Mary less available to help her family with arrangements, she misses several extra days of work. Her choice is ironic because, by driving, she greatly increases her odds of being hurt or even dying. Flying is still the safest form of travel available.

Len enjoys walking his dog. Unfortunately, Len also worries that he may have forgotten to lock the door when he leaves the house. More often than not, after he turns the first corner, he goes back to check the lock. Some days, he checks the doorknob four or five times. He feels almost panicked at the idea of someone breaking into his house. Len doesn't realise that he's overestimating two risks. First, although his *thoughts* tell him he probably left the door

What are the odds?

Any person's odds of dying from a particular event in any year are calculated by dividing that year's population by the number of deaths caused by that event in that year. Your lifetime odds of dying of a particular cause are calculated by dividing the odds in that one year by the life expectancy of a person born in that year.

On any given day, the odds of being struck by lightning are about 1 in 250 million, and the lifetime odds of being killed

- By a dog are about 1 in 700,000

- By a poisonous snake, lizard, or spider are about 1 in 700,000

- By a firearm are about 1 in 202

- In air or space transport are about 1 in 5,000

- In a road traffic accident are about 1 in 81

Notice how the actual odds don't match very well with what people fear. Many more people fear thunderstorms, snakes, spiders, and flying in airplanes than fear driving a car or being shot and killed. It doesn't make a lot of sense does it? Finally, you should note that your individual odds may vary. If you regularly stand out in thunderstorms, holding your golf clubs in the air, your chances of being struck by lightning are a little higher than average.

unlocked, *reality* says that he has never done that. Secondly, only a few break-ins have occurred in his neighbourhood in the past several years. The odds of a burglar plotting to rob Len's home during his 30-minute foray with the dogs are astronomically small.

Both Len and Mary spend too much time and effort avoiding facing their fears, and what they fear is unlikely to occur. Subject your fears to a reality test. Weigh the odds carefully.

Whenever possible, look up the statistical evidence relating to your fears. Unfortunately, you can't always find statistics that help you.

The following story shows how people overestimate the probability of a horrible outcome.

Dennis rudely grabs the pan from his wife, Linda. He snaps at her, 'I'll finish browning the meat. Just go and set the table.' His abrupt manner hurts Linda's feelings, but she knows how anxious he gets when they have guests. Dennis tightly grips the pan over the stove, watching the colour of the meat carefully. He feels irritable and anxious, convinced that the dinner will turn out badly. He frets that the meat is too tough and the vegetables look soggy from overcooking. The stress is contagious, and by the time the visitors arrive, Linda is sharing his worries.

What outcome does Dennis predict? Almost every time that he and Linda entertain, Dennis believes that the food that they prepare will be terrible, their guests will be horrified, and he'll be humiliated. The odds of this outcome can't be looked up in a table or a book. So how can Dennis assess the odds realistically? You or Dennis can ask the following *questions to recalculate the odds* and then write some answers:

- ✔ How many times have I predicted this outcome, and how many times has it actually happened to me?

- ✔ How often does this happen to people I know?

- ✔ If someone I know made this prediction, would I agree?

- ✔ Am I assuming that this will happen just because I fear that it will, or is there a reasonable chance that it will really happen?

- ✔ Do I have any experiences from my past that would suggest my dire prediction is unlikely to occur?

In Dennis's case, he realises that both he and his wife have never actually ruined a dinner, although he predicted it numerous times.

Furthermore, he questioned his second prediction that his guests would feel horrified if the dinner did turn out badly. He recalled that one time he and Linda went to a barbeque when the meat was burned to the extent that it was inedible. Everyone expressed genuine sympathy and shared stories about their own cooking disasters. They ended up ordering pizza and considered it one of the most enjoyable evenings they'd spent in a long time. The hosts, far from humiliated, basked in the glow of goodwill.

Working through worry scenarios

Yes, but you may be thinking, bad things do happen. Lightning strikes. Bosses hand out bad assessments. Planes crash. Some days are just bad-hair days. Ships sink. People trip over and get laughed at. Some lose their jobs. Lovers break up, and marriages end in divorce.

The world gives us plenty of reasons to worry. Recalculating the true odds often helps. But you're still stuck with 'What if?' What if your concern truly happens?

Small-beer scenarios

What do people worry about? Most of the time they worry about inconsequential, *small-beer scenarios*. In other words, outcomes that while unpleasant, hardly qualify as life threatening. Nevertheless, these small scenarios manage to generate remarkable amounts of stress, apprehension, and worry.

Check out what's worrying Gerald, Sam, Tricia, and Carol:

Gerald worries about many things. Mostly, he worries about committing a social blunder. Before parties, he agonises over what to wear. Will he look too dressed up or too casual? Will he know what to say? What if he says something stupid and people laugh? As you may imagine, Gerald feels miserable at social events. When he walks into a crowd, he feels as though a spotlight has turned his way and everyone in the room is staring at him. He imagines that people not only focus on him, but that they also judge him critically.

Sam worries as much as Gerald; he just has a different set of worries. Sam broods over the idea that he'll lose control and have to run away from wherever he is. If he's sitting in a classroom, he wonders whether he'll get so anxious that he'll have to leave, and of course he assumes everyone will know why he left and think that something is terribly wrong with him. If he's at a crowded shopping centre, he's afraid he'll 'lose it' and start screaming and running out of control.

Seventeen-year-old **Tricia** is preoccupied with the possibility that her current boyfriend will leave her someday. If her boyfriend is tired and in a bad mood, Tricia instantly assumes he's upset with her. If he arrives 15 minutes late, she figures he's been spending time with another girl. Not only does she assume he'll eventually leave her, but when he does, she can't imagine that life could go on without him.

Carol is a journalist. She feels anxiety almost every day. She feels pressure in her chest when each deadline approaches and dreads the day when she fails to get her story in on time. Making matters worse, she sometimes has writer's block and can't think of the next word to type for 15 or 20 minutes; all the while, the clock advances and the deadline nears. She's seen colleagues lose their jobs when they consistently fail to reach their deadlines, and she fears meeting the same fate one day. It's hard for Carol to stop thinking about her deadlines.

What do Gerald, Sam, Tricia, and Carol have in common? First, they all have considerable anxiety, stress, and tension. They worry almost every single day of their lives. They can't imagine the horror of dealing with the possibility of their fears coming true. But, more importantly, they worry about events that happen all the time and that other people manage to cope with when they do happen.

Gerald, Sam, Tricia, and Carol all underestimate their own ability to cope. What if Gerald spills something at a party and people around him notice? Would Gerald fall to the floor unable to move? Would people point and laugh at him? Not likely. He'd probably blush, feel embarrassed, and clean up the mess. The party and Gerald's life would go on. Even if a few rude people laugh at Gerald, most would forget the incident and certainly would not view Gerald any differently.

Carol, on the other hand, has a bigger worry. Her worst-case scenario involves losing her job. That sounds serious. What would she do if she lost her job? The following *coping questions* help Carol to discover her true coping resources. You can use these questions to help deal with your own worst fears.

1. Have I ever dealt with anything like this in the past?

2. How much will this affect my life a year from now?

3. Do I know anyone who has coped with something like this, and how did they do it?

4. Do I know anyone to whom I could turn for help or support?

5. Can I think of a creative new possibility that could result from this challenge?

Trying to come to terms with her fears, Carol writes her answers to these coping questions:

1. **No, actually I've never lost a job before.**

   The first question didn't help Carol discover her hidden coping resources, but it did help her see that possibly she was overestimating the risk of losing her job.

2. **If I did lose my job, I'd probably have some financial problems for a while, but I'm sure I could find another job.**

3. **Well, my friend Janet lost her job a few months ago.**

   She was on benefits for a bit and asked her parents for a little assistance. Now she has a new job that she really likes.

4. **I'd hate to have to ask, but my brother would always help me out if I really needed it.**

   Actually, come to think of it, it might balance our relationship a bit, as up to now I've always been the one there to support and help him.

5. **Well, when I think about it, I really hate these daily deadlines at the newspaper, so the job is not really right for me.**

   But I do have a teaching qualification. What with the shortage of teachers right now, I could always try to get a job teaching and have at least some time off in the holidays. Best of all, I could use the time off to write the novel I've always dreamed about writing. Maybe I'll hand in my notice now and do that!

It's amazing how often asking yourself these questions can *decatastrophise* your imagined worst-case scenario. Answering these questions can help you see that you can deal with the vast majority of your worries – or at least the small-beer ones.

But how about the worst-case scenarios? Could you cope with real disasters?

Worst-case scenarios

Some peoples' fears involve issues that go way beyond social embarrassment or temporary financial loss. Severe illness, death, terror, natural disasters, disfigurement, major disabilities, and loss of a loved one are worst-case scenarios. How would you possibly cope with one of these? We're not going to tell you it would be easy, because it wouldn't be.

Marilyn's mother and grandmother both died of breast cancer. She knows that her odds of getting breast cancer are higher than most people's. Almost every day of her adult life she worries about her health. She insists on monthly checkups, and every stomach upset, bout of fatigue, or headache becomes an imagined tumour.

Her stress concerns both her family and her doctor. First, her GP helps her to see that she is overestimating her risk. Unlike her mother and grandmother, Marilyn goes for yearly mammograms and performs regular self-examinations. Not only that, she exercises regularly and eats a much healthier diet than her mother or grandmother did.

But still, Marilyn realistically has an increased chance of getting breast cancer. How would she possibly cope with this worst-case scenario? You may be surprised to know that the same questions used to deal with the small-beer scenarios can help you deal with the worst-case scenarios. Take a look at how Marilyn answered our five coping questions:

Question: Have I ever dealt with anything like this in the past?

Marilyn's answer: Unfortunately, yes. I helped my mother when she was going for chemotherapy. It was horrible, but I do remember times when we laughed together. I understand that chemotherapy isn't nearly as bad as it used to be. I never felt closer to my mother than during that time. We talked through many important issues.

Question: How much will this affect my life a year from now?

Marilyn's answer: Well, if I do get breast cancer, it will have a dramatic affect on my life a year from now. I may still be in treatment or recovering from surgery. And the earlier a tumour's found, the greater the chance it can be successfully treated.

These first two questions focus Marilyn on the possibility of getting cancer. Even though she worries about cancer, the intensity of the anxiety has prevented her from ever contemplating how she would deal with cancer if it actually occurred. Although she certainly hates the thought of chemotherapy or surgery, after she imagines the possibility, she realises she could probably cope with it.

The more you avoid a fear, the more terrifying it becomes.

Question: Do I know anyone who has coped with something like this, and how did they do it?

Marilyn's answer: Of course, my mother died of breast cancer. But during the last three years of her life, she enjoyed each moment. She got closer to all her children and made many new friends. We had some especially good times, and did so many things together that we might never have got round to without this as the trigger.

Question: Do I know anyone to whom I could turn for help or support?

Marilyn's answer: I know of a cancer support group in town. And my husband and sister would do anything for me.

Question: Can I think of a creative new possibility that could result from this challenge?

Marilyn's answer: I never thought of cancer as a challenge, it was a curse. But I guess I realise now that I can choose to be anxious and worried about it or just take care of myself and live life to the full. If I do get cancer, I can hopefully help others like my mother did, and I'll use the time I have in a positive way. Besides, there's a good chance that I could beat cancer and, with medical advances, those chances improve all the time. Meanwhile, I'm going to make sure that I don't wait until my final days to get close to my family.

When you have anxiety about something dreadful happening, it's important to stop avoiding the end of the story. Go there. The more you avoid contemplating the worst, the bigger the fear gets. In our work, we repeatedly find that our clients come up with coping strategies for the worst-case scenario, even the big stuff. When people avoid grappling with their fears instead of becoming copers, they turn into victims.

George, for example, fears flying. He recalculates the risks of flying and realises they're low. He says, 'I know it's relatively safe and that helps a little, but it still scares me.' Recently, George got a promotion. Unfortunately for George, the new position requires considerable travel. George's worst nightmare is that the plane will crash. George asks himself our coping questions and answers them as follows:

- ✔ **Have I ever dealt with anything like this in the past?**

  No, obviously I've never been in a plane crash before.

- ✔ **How much will this affect my life a year from now?**

  Not much, I'd probably be dead!

✔ **Do I know anyone who has coped with something like this, and how did they do it?**

No. None of my friends, relatives, or acquaintances has ever been in a plane crash.

✔ **Do I know anyone to whom I could turn for help or support?**

Obviously not. I mean, what could they do?

✔ **Can I think of a creative new possibility that could result from this challenge?**

How? In the few minutes I'd have on the way down, it's doubtful that many creative possibilities would occur to me.

Hmmm. George didn't seem to get much out of our coping questions did he? These questions don't do much good for a small number of worst-case scenarios. For those situations, we have the *ultimate coping questions:*

1. What is it about this eventuality that makes you think you absolutely could not cope and could not possibly stand it?

2. Is it possible that you really could deal with it?

George answers:

1. Okay, I can imagine two different plane crashes. In one, the plane would explode and I probably wouldn't even know what happened. In the other, something would happen to the engine, and I'd experience several minutes of absolute terror. That's what I really fear.

2. Could I deal with that? I suppose I've never thought of that before; it seemed too scary to contemplate. If I really put myself in the plane, I'd probably be gripping the seat, maybe even screaming, but I guess it wouldn't last for long. I suppose I could stand almost anything for a short while. At least if I went down in a plane, I know that my family would be well taken care of. When I really think about it, as unpleasant as it seems, I guess I could deal with it. I'd have to.

Most people fear dying to some extent – even those with strong religious convictions (which can help) rarely welcome the thought. Nevertheless, death is a universal experience. Although most people would prefer a painless, quick exit during sleep, many deaths aren't as easy.

If you have a particular way of dying that frightens you, actively contemplating it works better than trying to block it out of your mind. If you face your fear, you're likely to discover that, like George, you can deal with and accept almost any eventuality.

If you find yourself getting exceptionally anxious or upset by such contemplation, professional help may be useful.

Cultivating Calm Thinking

Anxious thoughts capture your attention. They hold your reasonable mind hostage. They demand all your calmness and serenity as ransom. Thus, when you have anxious thoughts, it helps to pursue and destroy them by weighing the evidence, recalculating the odds, and reviewing your true ability to cope.

Another option is to overwhelm your anxious thoughts with calm thoughts. You can accomplish this by using one of two techniques. First, you can try what we call the friend perspective, or you can construct new, calm thoughts to replace your old, anxious thoughts.

Being your own best friend

Sometimes, simple strategies work wonders. This can be one of them. When your anxious thoughts hold most of your reasonable mind hostage, you still have a friend in reserve. Where? Within yourself.

Pick a worry. Any worry. Listen to that worry and everything outrageous it has to say to you. For example, **Roger** worries about his bills. He has a credit card balance of a few thousand pounds. His car insurance is coming up in a couple of weeks, and he doesn't have the money to pay for it. When Roger contemplates his worry, he thinks that maybe he'll be made bankrupt, his car will be repossessed, and that eventually, he'll lose his house. He feels he has no options and that his situation is hopeless. Roger loses sleep because of his worry. Anxiety shuts down his ability to reason and analyse his dilemma.

Now we ask Roger to help an old friend. We tell him to imagine that James, a friend of his, is sitting in a chair across from him. His friend is in a bit of a mess financially and needs advice on what to do. James fears he will lose everything if he can't come up with the money to pay his car insurance. We ask Roger to come up with some ideas for James.

Surprising to Roger, but not to us, Roger comes up with a whole host of good ideas. He tells James, 'Talk to your car insurers about monthly rather than annual payments. Also, you can possibly increase your limit on your credit card as a short-term solution. Isn't there also a chance of doing some over-time at work? Talk to a debt advisor. Can a friend or relative help out with a short-term loan? In the long run, you need to chip away at that credit-card debt and pull back a little on your spending.'

Another way in which you can use the best friend technique is a development of *cognitive therapy*, the therapy on which this book is based, called 'compassionate mind training'. Using this method, you learn to catch those critical voices (remember Marion's mother and Veronica's father?) and to identify the unpleasant and upsetting things others have said to you and that you now say to yourself.

Compassionate mind training involves providing counter-arguments to those critical thoughts you have about yourself. In the same way that hearing the horrible things others say about you makes you feel bad, saying positive, supportive, encouraging things to yourself, about yourself, can make you feel far better about yourself. You learn to say the helpful things to yourself with the full expression, emotion, and compassion that someone special and encouraging would use. You will usually find this has an even more powerful effect than just listing the counter-arguments against your negative thoughts. The arguments are so much more powerful, convincing, and meaningful if you can hear them caringly spoken in your imagination. Using this technique, rather than requiring the support to come from others, you can learn to be your own best friend.

Try this technique when you're all alone – alone, that is, except for your friend within.

Truly imagine that your good friend is sitting across from you and talk out loud. Take your time and really try to help. Brainstorm with your friend. You don't have to come up with instant or perfect solutions. Seek out any and every idea you can, even if it sounds foolish at first – it just may lead you to a creative solution.

This approach works because it helps you pull back from the overwhelming emotions that block good, reasonable thinking. Don't dismiss this strategy just because of its simplicity!

Creating calm

Another way to create calm thoughts is to simply look at your anxious thoughts and develop an alternative, more reasonable perspective. The key to this approach is to put your reasonable thoughts on paper. This exercise can have the same effect as chemical medication, but writing your reasonable thoughts down, rather than just thinking of them in your head, is like taking a stronger dose of the medicine and increasing its effectiveness.

This strategy doesn't equate with mere positive thinking, because if you simply create an alternative that has no logical backing to support it, it won't help. It's not enough to just contradict the disturbing thoughts – be sure that your reasonable perspective is something you can at least partially believe in. In other words, your emotional side may not fully buy in to your alternative view at first, but the new view should be something a reasonable person would find believable.

Your task will be easier if you have already subjected your anxious thinking to weighing the evidence, recalculating the odds, and re-evaluating your coping resources for dealing with your imagined worst-case scenarios.

In Table 5-3 are some examples of anxious thoughts and their reasonable alternatives. We also provide you with arguments that don't have any logical support and that we *don't* think are useful.

Table 5-3	Developing a Reasonable Perspective	
Anxious Thought	*Reasonable Alternative*	*Unsubstantiated Contradiction*
If I wear a tie and no-one else does, I'll look like an idiot.	If no-one else wears a tie, some people may notice. However, they probably won't make a big deal of it. Even if a couple of people do, it won't matter to me at all a few weeks from now.	Everyone will think I look great no matter what!
If I get a C in this exam, I'll be humiliated. I have to be at the top of my class. I couldn't stand it if I weren't.	If I get a C, I certainly won't be happy. But I'll still have a good overall average plus a good chance at a scholarship. I'll just work harder next time. I'd love to be at the top of my class, but life will go on just fine if I fall short of that.	There's no way that I won't get an A. I must, and I shall.
If I lose my job, in a matter of weeks I'll be bankrupt.	If I lose my job, it will cause some hardship. However, the odds are good that I'll find another one. And my wife has offered to increase her hours to help out if I need her to.	I could never lose my job!
I'd rather walk down 20 flights of stairs than take this lift. The thought of the doors closing terrifies me.	It's time I tackled this fear, because the odds of a lift crashing are infinitesimally small. Using the lift is pretty scary, but perhaps I can start by just going up or down a couple of floors and working my way up (or down) from there.	I'm not frightened of taking the lift to the top.

We show you the unsubstantiated or contradictory perspective because it's important not to go there. You may think the last example looks great. Just get over your fear in an instant. That would be nice, we suppose, if only it worked that way. The problem with that approach is that you can be setting yourself up for failure if you try it. Imagine someone truly terrified of lifts trying to jump in and take it to the top floor all at once. More likely than not, the person would do it that once, feel horror, and make the fear even worse.

Be gentle with yourself; go slowly when confronting your anxious thoughts and fears.

The ABC of CBT

Cognitive behavioural therapy (CBT) techniques have been developed from extensive research, and studies indicate that treatments based on CBT principles lead to the greatest long-term success. The principles underlying all the exercises in this book have come from the development of CBT.

CBT works on the principle that people's behaviour and emotions depend to a large degree on their perception of what they understand is happening. What we think and anticipate can greatly affect our reaction to events and people. Having understood what you are thinking and how to deal with your thoughts, it is possible to train yourself in a different way. This new behaviour can then lead to a potentially more satisfying way of life and become part of your normal lifestyle.

A helpful way to think about understanding and using CBT to overcome anxiety is that the crux of CBT is as straightforward as ABC.

- ✔ **A** refers to the *Antecedent*, or the trigger that sets you off in a direction you didn't want to go in.
- ✔ **B** is for the *Beliefs* that you then apply to the situation.
- ✔ **C** is for the *Consequences* – the outcome.

Learning your ABC goes like this:

1. **First, identify the trigger thought or feeling and call it A – the antecedent event.**
2. **Identify B – your belief about the antecedent.**
3. **Finally, identify C – the consequence of your belief. How did you act and emotionally or physically feel about the situation?**

As you've seen, it's beliefs that largely cause the stressful consequences, not necessarily the actual antecedent event itself. This explains why many people aren't stressed about meeting important deadlines, giving a presentation, or meeting new people – they believe they will cope well and don't predict any awful consequences.

A key part in the process of challenging beliefs is to question the demands that say you must, ought, should, or have to achieve a particular outcome. Ask yourself:

- Who says you have to believe certain things?
- Is it just you in your head or do others make these demands too?
- Are others necessarily infallible?
- What would happen if you did fail?
- Would it really be that unbearably awful?
- Are you exaggerating the outcome?

Think of how you could bear it, reminding yourself you don't have to like it. Challenge those over-generalisations – how does not meeting one target make you a total failure in everything? Isn't that a bit unfair on you – and would you judge others in this way?

The aim, having identified A, the antecedent, and challenged B, your beliefs about the antecedent, is to enable you to make your beliefs more realistic and flexible and less demanding, and no longer so absolute. When beliefs are modified, you find that you usually feel emotionally and physically different, and this enables you to evict catastrophising and its companion, procrastination, and get on with the task in hand.

It's very important to tell yourself that like any new skill, learning your ABC takes a while before you know it by rote and incorporate it automatically into your daily routine.

Think of learning your ABC as a daily mental workout – the gym for your mind, where you practise challenging unhelpful, anxiety-inducing thinking. Your workout strengthens you as you develop new stress-reducing, life-improving beliefs.

Chapter 6

Changing Your Anxiety – Provoking Assumptions

- -

- -

*D*riving in heavy traffic, disagreeing with the boss, travelling by air, paying bills, fighting with your partner, receiving a bad assessment, going to a job interview, making a speech, getting bad news from the doctor, or noticing that your flies are undone while leaving church may all make many people anxious. You may recognise one or several of these as situations that apply to you, while a few people aren't bothered by any of these, and indeed rarely become anxious at all. We don't expect they are reading this book, however.

This chapter explains why certain activities or events make you anxious, while others don't. You'll see how certain beliefs or assumptions generate excessive worry and anxiety. These beliefs come from your life experiences and are not signs of a failing on your part. Questionnaires help you discover which assumptions may upset you and create anxiety. We call these assumptions your *anxiety-provoking assumptions,* or APAs – the things that really stir you up. We provide ways for you to challenge those assumptions. Replacing your APAs with calming assumptions can substantially reduce your anxiety.

Understanding APAs

An assumption is something that you believe, without any question, is correct. You don't think about your assumptions; rather, you take them for granted as basic truths. For example, you probably believe that autumn follows summer, and that someone who smiles at you is friendly and someone who scowls at you isn't, at least most of the time. Therefore, your assumptions provide a map for getting you through life.

And that's not necessarily a bad thing. Your assumptions guide you through your days with less effort. For example, most people assume their salaries will be paid more or less on time. That assumption allows them to plan ahead, pay bills, and avoid unnecessary worry. If people didn't make this assumption, they'd constantly check with their payroll department or bosses to ensure timely payment, irritating all concerned.

Similarly, most people assume that food sold in the shops is safe to eat. Otherwise, they'd boil away germs and flavour to protect themselves from harm. They'd intensely scrutinise and test food they couldn't boil.

And when you go to the doctor, you probably assume your GP will provide good care and has your best interests at heart. Otherwise, you'd think twice before allowing any sort of medical examination.

Unfortunately, sometimes assumptions fail to provide useful, reality-based information. They may even distort reality so much that they give rise to considerable distress. For example, before giving a speech, you may tremble, quiver, and sweat. You worry that you may stumble over your words, drop your notes, or even worse, faint from fear. Even though very few, if any, of these things have actually happened in the past, you still keep assuming that the next time will be that total fiasco. That dread of being embarrassed comes from an APA.

Unquestioned beliefs that you hold on to, APAs, assume the worst about you or the world.

When activated, these beliefs cause anxiety and worry. Unfortunately, most people aren't even aware that they have these beliefs. Therefore, APAs can go unchallenged for many years, thus leaving them free to fuel anxiety.

Finding Your APAs

Perhaps you want to know whether you hold any APAs. People usually don't even know if they have these troubling beliefs, so they don't question them. Challenging APAs has to start with knowing which ones you have. In our work with clients, we found that five major APAs commonly trouble them:

- **Perfectionism:** Perfectionists assume they must do everything right or they will have failed totally and the consequences will be utterly devastating. They worry over minor details.

- **Approval:** Approval addicts assume they must win the approval of others at any cost to themselves. They can't stand criticism.

✔ **Vulnerability:** Those with the vulnerability assumption feel at the mercy of life's forces. They worry constantly about possible disasters.

✔ **Control:** Those with the control assumption feel that they can't trust or rely on anyone but themselves. They always want to be the driver, not the passenger.

✔ **Dependency:** Those with the dependency assumption feel they can't survive on their own and turn to others for help.

Assumptions have a powerful influence on the way that you respond to circumstances. Suppose, for example, that the majority of comments that you get during a performance review at work are quite positive, but one sentence describes a minor problem.

✔ If you have the perfectionism assumption, you severely criticise yourself for your failure. You won't even see the positive comments.

✔ If you have the approval assumption, you worry about whether your boss still likes you.

✔ On the other hand, the vulnerability assumption leads you to believe that you're about to lose your job, then your house and car, and finally your partner and children.

✔ By contrast, if you have a control assumption, you focus on why others couldn't get their bit right – it wouldn't have been a problem if you'd been in charge of it all.

✔ Finally, if you have the dependency assumption, you look to others for support and help. You may discover that you have the perfect solution to the problem, but you run it by several people, several times over, to get their approval for it.

Same event, but various individuals react completely differently depending on which assumption they hold. Just imagine the reaction of someone who simultaneously holds several of these assumptions. One sentence in a performance review could set off a huge emotional storm of anxiety and distress.

You may have one or more of these assumptions to one degree or another. We have a quiz for you to take to see which, if any, APAs you hold.

Testing Your Beliefs and Assumptions

In Table 6-1, place a tick in the column marked T if a statement is true or mostly true as a description of you; conversely, place a tick in the column marked F if a statement is false or mostly false as a description of you. Please don't mark your statement as T or F simply based on how you think you should be, but rather on the basis of how you think you really do act and respond to events in your life.

Table 6-1		The APAs Quiz
T	*F*	***Perfectionism***
		If I'm not good at something, I'd rather not do it.
		When I make a mistake, I feel terrible.
		I think that if something's worth doing, it's worth doing perfectly.
		I can't stand to be criticised.
		I don't want to hand in my work to anyone until it's perfect.
T	*F*	***Approval***
		I often worry about what other people think.
		I sacrifice my needs to please others.
		I hate speaking in front of a group of people.
		I need to be nice all the time or people won't like me.
		I can rarely say no to people.
T	*F*	***Vulnerability***
		I worry about things going wrong.
		I worry a great deal about my safety, health, and finances.
		Many times, I feel like a victim of circumstances.
		I worry a great deal about the future.
		I feel pretty helpless much of the time.
T	*F*	***Control***
		I hate taking orders from anyone.
		I like to be involved in everything.
		I hate to leave my fate in the hands of others.
		Nothing would be worse than losing control.
		I do much better as a leader than a follower.

T	F	Dependency
		I'm nothing unless someone loves me.
		I could never be happy on my own.
		I ask advice about most things that I do.
		I need a great deal of reassurance.
		I rarely do things without other people.

Most people endorse one or more of these items as true. So don't worry too much if you found quite a few statements that apply to you. For example, who doesn't hate worrying about money? And most people worry at least a little about the future.

So how do you know if one of these assumptions causes a problem for you? You start by looking at the assumptions, one at a time. If you ticked one or more items as true, that raises the possibility that this assumption causes you some trouble. Just how much trouble depends on how much distress you feel.

Laura Smith, one of the authors of _Overcoming Anxiety For Dummies,_ battled with the vulnerability assumption. She writes, 'One evening I was sitting in the beauty salon. Suddenly, a thug stormed in, demanding that everyone lie on the floor and hand over their money and jewellery. He brandished a hand-gun to emphasise his point. Not long after the incident, I realised that I had acquired the APA of vulnerability. I found myself worrying about my safety much more than I had in the past. I started to nervously scan car parks for miscreants and jumped at loud noises. When I found myself waking up from nightmares, I knew that the vulnerability assumption was creating trouble and that I needed to do something about it. I used some of the techniques described in Chapter 8. These strategies included gradually returning to the scene of the crime, talking about the crime, and relaxation. Soon, I found my vulnerability assumption abating.'

Ask yourself what makes you feel especially anxious, and does it have to do with one or more items that you checked as true? If so, you probably struggle with that particular APA.

If you have a number of these APAs, don't have a go at yourself! It's likely that you developed your APAs for good reasons. And you should rather congratulate yourself for starting to figure out the problem. That's the first step towards feeling better.

Suffering a Spell of APAs

If you have too much anxiety, one or more APAs undoubtedly cause you problems. But it's especially important to know that you're not crazy for having APAs. That's because people acquire these assumptions in two completely understandable ways:

- ✔ When shocking, traumatic events shatter previously held assumptions
- ✔ When experiences in childhood prevent the development of a reasonable sense of safety, security, acceptance, or approval

Having your reasonable assumptions shattered

The following example illustrates how life can create an APA:

Bill had always assumed, like most people do, that a green light signals that it's safe to proceed through a junction. Bill drove for 20 years without mishap. One day on the way to work, Bill drove through a junction that he'd safely crossed hundreds of times before. Suddenly, a 4 x 4 jumped the red light and slammed into the side of Bill's hatchback. Bill sustained serious injuries but recovered.

When Bill returned to driving, he found himself slowing down and crawling across junctions with intense feelings of anxiety. He could barely make himself drive to work and back each day and avoided driving whenever possible. Bill's doctor tells him he now has high blood pressure and that he needs to reduce his stress. Bill worries about his worry but doesn't know what he can do about it.

Bill has formed a new assumption – an APA. The vulnerability assumption plagues him. He now worries that driving is dangerous and requires the utmost vigilance. Bill had good reason to form that assumption, and Bill's belief, like most APAs, contains a grain of truth in that driving can be dangerous. However, as with all APAs, the problem lies in the fact that Bill overestimates the dangers of driving. Therefore, he feels excessive anxiety whenever he gets into the car.

Bill's anxiety didn't emerge until he was an adult, but anxiety can begin at any age. Many adopt their APAs in childhood.

Cars: A dangerous mode of transport?

Although Bill now overestimates the risks of driving, it's true that driving does involve some significant dangers. Comparing travel on buses, planes, trains, and cars, deaths from car accidents far exceed deaths from all these other modes of transport combined. Sounds scary, doesn't it? However, the odds of dying in your car don't look all that bad. For every 100 million miles driven, less than one fatality occurs.

Acquiring assumptions in childhood

You may have been one of the lucky ones who glided through childhood feeling loved, accepted, safe, and secure. Perhaps you lived in a four-bedroom house in leafy suburbia, with two loving parents, a brother, and a sister, and never a cross word was spoken. Or maybe not. You probably didn't have a perfect childhood. Not many do. For the most part, your parents probably did the best they could, but they were human. Perhaps they had bad tempers or maybe ran into financial difficulties. Or possibly they had addictions or they failed to look out for your safety as well as they should have. For these and numerous other reasons, you may have acquired one or more APAs.

Unlike Bill, **Harold** didn't have to wait until adulthood to suffer from his APA. Harold's mother rarely gave him much approval. She harshly criticised almost everything he did. For example, his room was never clean enough and his exam results were never good enough. Even when he brought his mother a gift, she told him it was the wrong colour or size. He felt he could do almost nothing right.

Slowly but surely, Harold acquired an APA – 'I must be absolutely perfect, or I will be a total failure'. Being perfect is pretty hard. So you can imagine why he now feels anxious most of the time. And a bit like Boxer, the horse in George Orwell's novel *Animal Farm,* Harold sees the solution to each setback as being 'I must try harder'. But that solution ultimately failed for Boxer – he died of a heart attack, brought on by overwork – and that solution is likely to fail for Harold too in the long run.

If you have APAs, you don't question them. You believe in them wholeheartedly. Just as he assumes the sky is blue, Harold believes that he's either perfect or a complete failure. When Harold undertakes a project, he feels intense anxiety due to his morbid fear of making a mistake. Harold's APA is that of painful perfectionism and it makes him miserable, but he doesn't know why.

Challenging Those Unhelpful Assumptions: Running a Cost/Benefit Analysis

Now you have a better idea about which APAs may be giving you trouble. In the old days, many therapists would have told you that insight is enough. We disagree. Pretend you just took an eye test and found out that you suffer from severe short-sightedness. Wow, you have insight! But what does that change? Not much. You still walk around bumping into the furniture.

You're about to get a prescription for seeing through your problematic assumptions. It starts with a *cost/benefit analysis*. To make such an analysis, you simply add up the value of the benefits of a course of action and subtract the costs associated with it. This analysis paves the way for making changes.

Perhaps you think that your painful perfectionism assumption is good and appropriate. Maybe you believe that you have profited from your perfectionism and that it has helped you accomplish more in your life. If so, why in the world would you want to challenge or change it? The answer is simple. You wouldn't.

Therefore, you need to take a cold, hard look at the costs as well as any possible benefits of perfectionism. Only if the costs outweigh the benefits does it make sense to do something about your perfectionism. Take a look at Pat, a painful perfectionist.

Pat the perfectionist

Pat, a successful barrister, works about 70 hours per week. Her cupboard is full of power suits; she wears her perfectionism like a badge of honour. Pat works out to maintain her trim figure and manages to attend all the right social events. At 43 years of age, Pat stands at the top of her profession. Too busy for a family of her own, she dotes on her nine-year-old niece and gives her lavish birthday and Christmas presents. Pat is shocked when her doctor tells her that her blood pressure is sky high. Her doctor wonders about the stress in her life. Pat says that it's nothing that she can't handle. Her doctor enquires about Pat's sleep habits, and she replies, 'What sleep?'

Pat is in big trouble and she doesn't even know it. She believes that her high income is due to her unremittingly high standards and that she can't let up in the slightest way. Take a look at Pat's cost/benefit analysis of perfectionism.

A cost/benefit analysis starts with listing every conceivable benefit of an APA. Including every benefit your imagination can possibly conjure up is important. Then, and only then, should you start thinking about the costs of the assumption. Once again, include any and every benefit that you can imagine. Take a look at Table 6-2 to see what Pat wrote in defence of her perfectionism.

Table 6-2	Cost/Benefit Analysis of Pat's Painful Perfectionism	
Benefits	*Costs*
My income is higher because of my perfectionism.	
I rarely make mistakes.	
I'm widely respected for my work.	
I always dress professionally and look good.	
Other people admire me.	
I'm a role model for my niece.	

Pat's attachment to her perfectionism is no small wonder. Filling out the benefits in her cost/benefit analysis (see Table 6-2) is easy for her, but what about the costs? Pat will probably have to put in much more effort and work to complete the costs, and she may even have to ask other people for ideas. Now, review in Table 6-3 what she wrote after she worked at the task and consulted others.

Table 6-3	Cost/Benefit Analysis of Pat's Painful Perfectionism	
Benefits	*Costs*
My income is higher because of my perfectionism.	I don't have much time for fun.
I rarely make mistakes.	I'm anxious and maybe that's why my blood pressure is running so high.
I'm widely respected for my work.	I don't have many friends.
I always dress professionally and look good.	I spend huge amounts of time and money on clothes and makeup.

(continued)

Table 6-3 *(continued)*

Benefits	Costs
Other people admire me.	I get very irritable when people don't measure up.
I'm a role model for my niece.	Some people hate me for my uncompromising standards and high expectations of them. I've lost several secretaries in the last six months.
	I hardly ever see my niece because I'm so busy.
	Sometimes I drink too much to unwind.
	Actually, I think that my focus on work has kept me from finding a meaningful relationship.

Don't get anxious about how you'll manage to prepare your own cost/benefit analysis. Read the following examples; they give you some good ideas. Then we give you some simple guidelines.

The cost/benefit analysis helps you to decide if you really want to challenge your APAs. You would probably agree that Pat's example shows more costs than benefits. But wait, it isn't finished. The final step is to examine carefully whether you would indeed lose all the benefits by changing the assumption.

For example, Pat attributes her high income to her dedication and long working hours. Perhaps she's partly right, but would her income totally evaporate if she worked just a little less? If she worked less, her income would probably drop a bit, but with less anxiety, she may increase her efficiency enough to make up the difference. If she were less irritable, she would be able to retain her secretarial staff and gain efficiency once again. And would Pat actually start making more mistakes if she relaxed her standards? Research suggests that excessive anxiety actually decreases performance. With respect to her niece, Pat isn't really giving the benefit that she thinks she is, because she's not around enough to serve as an effective role model. Finally, more people fear Pat than admire her.

So, you see, many times the perceived benefits of an assumption can evaporate on closer inspection.

Anxiety: How much is too much?

A little bit of anxiety seems to improve performance and reduce mistakes. Some anxiety channels attention to the task at hand. However, when perfectionism reaches extreme levels, so does anxiety, and performance drops off. Excessive anxiety interferes with the ability to recall previously learned information, and mistakes multiply. If you draw it on a graph, there's an inverted U shape between anxiety and performance. Initially, low anxiety and poorer performance go together. Then as anxiety increases (along the horizontal axis of the graph), so does the level of performance, which rises higher up the vertical axis. However, after a certain point, the greater your anxiety gets, the worse your performance becomes, as the inverted U drops down to lower and lower levels.

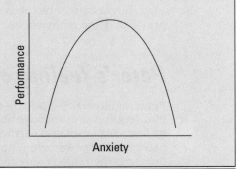

Anne's approval addiction

Anne craves approval and abhors the idea of rejection. Anne, a postgraduate social work student, has to meet weekly with her manager for supervision of her casework. She dreads those supervision sessions, always fearing her manager's criticism.

Anne does a huge amount for her clients; she would do anything that she thinks they may need help with, and spends hours of her own time, even running errands for them if they ask. Her manager tries to tell her to cut down on the excessive help she is giving to her clients. He says that when she bends over backwards to assist her clients, it doesn't actually help her or them. She cries after hearing her manager's comments.

However, Anne's worst fears concern the presentations she has to make to the other social work trainees on her course. Before giving these, she spends huge amounts of time in the bathroom, feeling utterly nauseous. During lively class discussions, Anne remains quiet, and almost never takes sides. Anne is addicted to approval.

Anne walks quietly through life. People rarely criticise her. She avoids embarrassment by not taking risks. She is kind-hearted and people like her. What's wrong with that?

Well, a cost/benefit analysis of Anne's APA, in particular her addiction to approval (see the bulleted list in the section 'Finding Your APAs', earlier in this chapter), reveals that people walk all over her. It also shows that fellow students fail to appreciate how bright she is, because she rarely speaks up in class. Anne neglects her own needs and at times feels resentful when she does so much for others and they do so little in return. Anne's approval addiction doesn't give her what she expects. Sure, she rarely receives criticism, but because she takes so few risks, she never gets the approval and praise that she really wants.

Peter's feeling of vulnerability

Peter, a university graduate with a business degree, receives a promotion that requires him to move abroad to California, but he turns it down because he fears big cities and earthquakes. Peter watches the weather channel and listens to the news before he ventures any distance from home, and avoids driving if the radio reports any chance of bad weather. Peter's worry restricts his life. He also worries about his health and often visits his doctor, complaining of vague symptoms such as nausea, headaches, and fatigue. Peter's doctor suggests that his worry may be causing many of his physical problems. She tells Peter to fill out a cost/benefit analysis of his anxiety-provoking vulnerability assumption. Table 6-4 represents Peter's efforts.

Table 6-4	Cost/Benefit Analysis of Peter's Vulnerability Assumption
Benefits	*Costs*
I keep myself safe.	I worry all the time.
I work hard to stay healthy.	Sometimes I can't stop thinking about my health.
I stay away from harm.	I'm so concerned about getting hurt that I've never enjoyed what other people do, such as skiing or trips abroad, let alone considered living overseas.
I am more careful than most about saving for retirement.	I worry so much about tomorrow that I forget to enjoy today.
I don't take unnecessary risks.	My doctor tells me that my worry probably harms my health more than anything else.

Someone as entrenched as Peter in his anxiety-provoking vulnerability assumption certainly isn't going to give it up just because of his cost/benefit analysis. However, this analysis starts the ball rolling by showing him that his assumption is very costly indeed. The exercise motivates him to start thinking about doing something different.

Geoff's need for control

Geoff, the head of a division at his engineering company, likes order in his life. His employees know him as a taskmaster who micro-manages, constantly intervening in their work. Geoff takes pride in the fact that, although he asks for plenty, he demands more of himself than he does of his employees. He issues orders and expects immediate results. His division leads the company in productivity.

You may think that Geoff has it made. It certainly sounds like his issue with control pays off handsomely. But scratch the surface and you see a different picture. Although known for productivity, his division is viewed as lacking in creativity and leads all others in requests for transfers. The real cost of Geoff's control assumption comes crashing down upon him when at 46 years of age, he suffers his first heart attack.

Geoff has spent many years feeling stressed and anxious, but he never looks closely at the issue. Geoff's quest for control leads to the opposite of what he wanted. Ultimately, he loses control of his life and health.

If control is one of your APAs, do a cost/benefit analysis. Geoff's fate doesn't have to be yours too.

Daniel's dependency

Daniel lived with his parents until, at 31 years of age, he married Dorothy. He met Dorothy through his church singles group and decided immediately to marry her. Dorothy seemed independent and secure, qualities that Daniel craved but lacked. At the beginning of their relationship, Dorothy enjoyed and was flattered by Daniel's constant attention. Today, he still calls her at work three or four times every day, asking for advice about small, inconsequential matters and sometimes seeking reassurance that she still loves him. If she's five minutes late, he's beside himself. He often worries that she'll leave him. Dorothy's friends tell her they aren't sure that Daniel can go to the toilet by himself. Daniel believes he can't survive without her.

We give an example of a cost/benefit analysis for Daniel in Table 6-5.

Table 6-5	Cost/Benefit Analysis of Daniel's Dependency Assumption
Benefits	*Costs*
I get people to help me when I need it.	I never find out how to handle difficult problems, tasks, situations, and people.
Other people take care of me.	Sometimes people resent having to take care of me.
Life is not as scary when I have someone to lean on.	My wife hates me calling her all the time.
It's not my fault when problems arise or plans don't work out.	My wife gets angry when I don't take initiative.
I'm never lonely because I always make sure that I have someone around.	I may drive my wife away if I continue to cling to her so much.
It makes life easier when someone else is in charge.	Sometimes I'd like to take care of something, but I think I'll screw it up.
	I haven't discovered how to master very much. Sometimes I feel like I haven't really grown up.

Someone like Daniel is unlikely to give up his unhelpful dependency assumption without more work than this. However, a cost/benefit analysis can provide an initial impetus. Meaningful change takes time and work.

Challenging your own APAs

You can run your own cost/benefit analysis. See the list of APAs in the 'Finding Your APAs' section, earlier in this chapter. Which ones trouble you? If you haven't already taken the APAs quiz in Table 6-1, earlier in this chapter, do so now and look at your answers. Do you tend towards perfection, vulnerability, control, dependency, or seeking approval?

First, if just one APA applies to you, select that one. Then, using the format of Table 6-5 as an example, fill out all the benefits that you can think of for your APA in the left-hand column. Fill in the costs in the right-hand column. If you get stuck, ask a trusted friend or partner for help. Seeking help when you have had a go but then find yourself stuck doesn't necessarily mean that you operate on the dependency assumption or that you're overly dependent. Refer to the cost/benefit analyses that Pat, Peter, and Daniel (refer to Tables 6-3, 6-4, and 6-5, respectively) filled out earlier in the chapter.

When you've finished your cost/benefit analysis, take another look at each of the benefits. Ask yourself whether those benefits will truly disappear if you change your APA. Pat the perfectionist believes that her income is higher because of her perfectionism, but is that really true? Many people report that they make far more mistakes when they feel under pressure. Perfectionism, if nothing else, certainly causes pressure. So, as a general rule, it's probably not the case that perfectionists earn more money and make fewer mistakes. More often than not, they end up not doing as well as they could, because their perfectionism leads them into making more mistakes, most especially in relation to their health. In certain professions, perfectionist tendencies could be advantageous, but when they begin to actually interfere with work and life outside work they become a problem. When you look carefully at your perceived benefits, you're likely to find, like Pat, that the presumed benefits will not evaporate if you change your assumption.

Similarly, Anne thinks she avoids embarrassment by never speaking in class. But she finds herself even more frightened and embarrassed when she's required to present in class than if she took more risks earlier. Avoiding what she fears seems to increase her worries. So Anne receives a double dose of what she so desperately wants to avoid.

APAs often get you the *opposite* of what you want.

APAs cause worry and stress and rarely give you any true benefits. If you're going to give up your assumptions, you'll need to replace them with a more balanced perspective.

Designing Balanced Assumptions

So, do you think you have to be perfect or that everyone has to like you all the time? Do you always need to be in charge? Do you feel that you can't manage life on your own? Or do you sometimes feel that the world is a dangerous place? These are the APAs that stir up worry, stress, and anxiety.

Another problem with these assumptions is that they do contain a kernel of truth. For example, it *is* nice when people like you, and it *is* nice to be in charge sometimes. We all need to depend on others sometimes as well. That sliver of truth makes people reluctant to abandon their assumptions. It's the old fear of not wanting to throw the baby out with the bathwater.

The solution is to find new, balanced assumptions that hold even greater truth – but old assumptions are like habits, and they're hard to break. To do so requires finding a new habit to replace the old. It also takes plenty of practice and self-control, but it isn't that difficult. We'll show you how to do it. You just need a little persistence.

We go over each of the assumptions and help you to see how to formulate an alternative more reasonable assumption to replace your old one. Try using these reasonable, balanced perspectives to argue with your APAs when they occur. Finally, when you develop a new assumption, try acting in ways that are consistent with that new belief, even if you don't fully subscribe to it yet. It's crucial that you behave *as if* the new assumptions are true, before you feel fully convinced. Research has shown that behaviour changes first, and feelings and beliefs then follow. So start acting the part (go for an Oscar) and later you will find that you no longer need to act the role – you have become that person, and it really *is* the new you.

Scaling down perfectionism

Perfectionists believe they have to be the best in everything they do. They feel horrible when they make mistakes and, if they're not outstanding at something, they'll generally refrain from trying it at all. Fortunately, a good cost/benefit analysis can often help them to see that perfectionism exacts a terrible toll.

But if not perfect, then what? Some people think it would mean going to the other extreme. Thus, if not perfect, these people assume that they would become total slobs with no standards at all.

 If you're worried about giving up on your perfectionism assumption, we have good news for you. The alternative is not the other extreme! You may find it helpful to copy the following statements, which are what we call 'balanced views', on an index card. Alternatively, you may want to think of your own statements. Just be sure they aim for the middle ground. Carry your card around with you as a reminder for when you start to get hung up on perfectionism.

- ✔ I like to do well at things, but it's unrealistic to think that I have to be the best at everything.

- ✔ I'll never be good at everything, and sometimes it's really fun just to try something new.

- ✔ Everyone makes mistakes; I need to deal with that fact when I make a mistake.

The deadly secrets of perfectionism

Perfectionism pays off . . . sometimes. A little bit of perfectionism can probably improve the quality of your work, sports, and other endeavours as long as you don't let it get out of hand. How bad is it when perfectionism gets too extreme? Worse than you may think. Perfectionists often become extreme procrastinators just to avoid making mistakes. Not only that, perfectionists more often develop obsessive-compulsive disorder (see Chapter 2), various types of anxiety disorders, depression, physical ailments, and eating disorders. Worst of all, it appears that adolescents who have a problem with perfectionism have a higher rate of suicide. So all the more reason to cut down on damaging perfectionist behaviour.

In other words, if you currently assume that you must be perfect and do everything right or you've failed totally, try to think in less extreme terms. A more balanced assumption would be that you like doing things well, but that *everyone make mistakes and so do you*. Can you really expect to be above the rest of us? *Collect evidence* that refutes your perfectionist assumption. For example, think about all the people you admire, yet who make numerous mistakes over time. When they make mistakes, do you suddenly see them as totally useless? Doubtful. Use the same standard for yourself.

Just try this one for size. 'If a job's worth doing, it's worth doing – even badly!'

'What?' perfectionists shriek in real terror. Well, in most of our day-to-day activities, they're wrong. Your car is absolutely filthy. You only have 15 minutes before you have to go out in it. Is it better to give it a lick and a promise – at least clean the front and back windscreens so you can see out – or to leave it covered in muck, because there's no point in starting a job that know you haven't the time to do perfectly? The answer's pretty obvious, we think – clean it, and get to see where you're going. Obviously, this doesn't apply to certain tasks; we wouldn't expect such latitude in your professional behaviour. Let's face it, for a brain surgeon to say an operation is 'good enough' and 'will do' just isn't good enough, and certainly won't do at all.

Balancing for an approval addict

Approval addicts desperately want to be liked all the time. They sacrifice their own needs in order to please others. Standing up for themselves is hard, because to do so would risk offending someone. When criticised, even unfairly, they tend to feel they are falling to pieces.

But isn't it good to want people's approval? As with all APAs, it's a matter of degree. Taken too far, the approval assumption can ruin your life.

But if you quit worrying about getting people's approval, what will happen then? Will you end up isolated, rejected, and alone? Is rudeness and selfish behaviour the alternative to being nice all the time?

If you worry about giving up on your approval addiction, we have a palatable alternative, and you just may want to carry these ideas in your pocket or handbag. Feel free to make some up on your own as well.

- ✔ What other people think matters, but it's not usually crucial.

- ✔ Some people won't like me no matter what I do. That's true for everyone.

- ✔ I need to start paying attention to my needs at least as much as to those of other people.

In addition, consider *collecting evidence* that refutes your approval addiction assumption. For example, think about people who you like and admire who manage to speak their minds and look out for their own needs. Why do you like them? It's probably not because they bow and scrape and indulge your every whim. Besides, someone who did that would probably put you right off.

If you feel addicted to approval and assume you must have the approval of others at all times and at virtually any cost, consider a more balanced perspective. Sure, everyone likes to be liked, but you need to realise that no matter what you do, some people won't like you some of the time. And some, if a personality clash occurs, may never like you, irrespective of what you do or don't do, because of their own prejudices.

Elaine, one of the authors of this book, vividly recalls a particularly difficult period in her life. Difficulties kept arising with a certain colleague. Not having experience with people who openly didn't like her, Elaine's reaction was to try to be nicer. But this colleague had particular prejudices, in particular towards people who were 'nice'. So the more angry the colleague became, the nicer Elaine tried to be, and you can see how this just exacerbated the situation. Years later, having learned and understood how to recognise and deal with the assumption that she needed approval, Elaine realises that what she should have done was to identify the personality clash and accept that she would never have the colleague's approval, but that they could work together without liking each other.

We suggest that you experiment with thinking that your needs matter, and that what other people think of you does not define your worth, and then try to act to meet your needs. Ensure your behaviour is now in line with these new beliefs – even if you don't yet fully believe them. We predict that you are likely to be pleasantly surprised by the outcome – Elaine certainly has been!

Balancing vulnerability

People who hold the vulnerability assumption feel unsafe and worry constantly about every conceivable mishap. They may worry about safety, health, natural disasters, or the future; they often feel like victims of life's circumstances. They feel helpless to do much about their lot.

People with this assumption fail to understand that worry never stopped a single catastrophe. Nor does excessive worry help you prepare for the inevitable bad luck and misfortune that occur in everyone's life.

However, a better alternative assumption can keep you reasonably safe, and without all that worry. If you want to give up your vulnerable assumption, try carrying these ideas with you and referring to them when you find yourself in danger of wobbling:

- ✔ I need to take reasonable precautions but stop constantly worrying about safety. There's only a limited amount of advance preparation that I or anyone else can put into practice.

- ✔ I will go to the doctor for an annual check up, pay attention to nutrition and exercise, and after that, worrying about my health is pointless.

- ✔ Some unfortunate mishaps are unforeseen and out of my control. I need to accept that bad things happen; worry is no shield. I'll deal with mishaps if and when they happen.

Again, if you hold the vulnerability assumption and feel that you're at the mercy of life's dangerous forces, you may want to consider a more balanced point of view. Try thinking that no-one can prevent the trials and tribulations of life, but that you can usually cope when they do occur. Collect evidence about the many unpleasant incidents that you were able to cope with in the past. For example, when you had high blood pressure, perhaps you exercised or took medication to control it, or when you lost someone that you cared for, you grieved but you survived.

Relaxing control

Some people always want to take charge. They can't stand taking orders. When in a group, they dominate the conversation. They always want to know everything that's going on around them in their families and at work. They don't delegate well. Some fear flying because they aren't in the cockpit.

Being a control freak is tiring and causes plenty of anxiety too. Perhaps you have trouble with this APA. Many highly successful, intelligent people do, and this assumption isn't easy to give up, but the costs to health, wellbeing, and relationships are staggering.

As for all APAs, we have an alternative balanced view that will serve you better than control ever did. Review our suggestions. And if you must take control and rewrite them, that's okay too!

- ✔ I can usually trust other people to do what they need to do. I don't have to manage everyone, and they're likely to resent me if I do.

- ✔ Asking for help or delegating a task isn't the end of the world, and sometimes delegating is much more efficient.

- ✔ I don't have to know every single detail of what's going on in order to feel and be in charge. Letting go reduces stress.

- ✔ Letting others lead can make them feel better and reduce the load on me.

- ✔ Sometimes it can even be fun to let others plan nice surprises.

Diminishing dependency

People with the anxiety-provoking dependency assumption believe they can't make it on their own. They ask for advice when they don't really need it and seek constant reassurance that they're loved or that what they've done is right. The thought of not having a close relationship terrifies them. They can barely imagine trying to live life alone. You're not likely to find someone with an anxiety-provoking dependency assumption eating alone in a restaurant. If they've gone to a conference, they will often order dinner in their rooms rather than sit at tables on their own.

Many APAs ironically backfire. Excessively dependent people eventually annoy and irritate those they depend on. Partners of dependent people often distance themselves from the relationships after they become weary of constant clinging and helplessness.

If you battle with dependency, consider some of our alternative thoughts. Write these on an index card and keep them handy for frequent review. Feel free to embellish these or come up with some of your own. Preferably, don't ask someone to help you with this task or to review and approve your efforts!

- ✔ It's nice to have someone who loves me, but I can survive on my own and have done so in the past.

- ✔ Seeking advice can be useful; working through an issue on my own is satisfying.

- ✔ I prefer to be with other people, but I can find out how to appreciate time alone.

- ✔ Usually others don't come up with anything I haven't already considered.

If you buy in to the unhelpful dependency assumption that you can't be all right on your own and that you need help with all that you do, try thinking in a more reasonable fashion. Realise that it's nice to have someone to depend on, but that you're capable of many independent actions. Collect evidence on your capabilities. Do you put petrol in your own car? Do you manage your own bank account? Do you get to work and back on your own? Can you remember the times that you did well without someone? Realising that you have taken independent action successfully and remembering that you have pulled yourself through a difficult time all by yourself can boost your confidence enough to take more independent action in the future.

If you find that your APAs rule your life and cause you intense anxiety and misery, you may want to consult a professional psychologist or mental health practitioner. But first, start with your GP to rule out physical causes. Sometimes anxiety does have a physical base, and your GP can give you a referral after physical causes have been excluded. Should you consult a professional, you'll still find this book useful, because most anxiety experts are familiar with the tools that we provide, and they'll help you implement them.

Above All: Be Kind to Yourself!

In our work with clients, we found that these APAs are surprisingly common, and many successful people who don't even have a full-blown anxiety disorder tend to fall under the influence of one or more of these assumptions. Therefore, it's important that you don't beat yourself up for being 'under the influence'.

The origins of your belief may be in your childhood or the result of a traumatic event. Possibly your parents were highly critical and that caused you to crave approval. Perhaps you had an unfortunate accident or trauma that caused you to feel vulnerable. Maybe your parents failed to provide you with consistent care and love, leading you to feel insecure and, as a result, you yearn for help and affection. These represent merely a few of an infinite number of explanations for why you may develop APAs. The point is that you didn't ask for your assumptions, and you came by them honestly. But be aware you don't have to be their victim in the future.

You have started on the road to overcoming anxiety. However, go slowly; take pleasure in the journey and realise that change takes time and practice. The most important three letters at this point in your journey are TTT – Things Take Time. Be patient with yourself.

Chapter 7

Watching Out for Worry Words

I'll never get this right . . . I always stumble over my words . . . I should really lose some weight . . . Nothing suits me . . . I look an utter mess . . . How can I be so stupid? . . . It will be terrible if I don't get that pay rise . . . I must get this finished, or I'll be in big trouble . . . What if I fail? . . . I'm totally useless at sport.

Imagine inner conversations like these. How would you feel talking to yourself like this? Probably not very good. This chapter explains how words alone can stir up a whirlwind of anxiety. We help you discover worry words to look out for. They come in several forms and categories, and you'll see how to track them down. Then we give you alternative words and phrases to calm your anxiety.

Getting to Grips with Worry Words

'Sticks and stones may break my bones, but words will never hurt me.' Perhaps you heard this saying as a child. Parents often try to make their children feel better by teaching them this retort to use when others have said nasty things to them. But it usually doesn't work, because words do have power. Words can frighten, judge, and hurt.

If those words only came from other people, that would hurt enough. But the words that you use to describe yourself, your world, your actions, and your future may have an even greater impact on you than what you hear from others.

At breakfast, a little worried about her husband's blood pressure, **Jeremy's wife Beverly** mentions that it looks like he's gained a little weight. 'Oh, really?' Jeremy queries. 'Maybe a little; but it's no big deal.' 'I just worry about your health', she replies.

A simple conversation between husband and wife. Or is it? Now, see what Jeremy thinks to himself about her comment over the course of the next few hours. 'I'm a *pig* . . . She's *totally disgusted* with me . . . She'll *never* want to have sex with me again . . . Losing weight is *impossible* for me . . . I'm *certain* that she'll leave me; that would be *unbearable.*'

By the afternoon, Jeremy feels intense anxiety and tension. He's so upset that he withdraws from Beverly and sulks through the rest of the day. Beverly knows that something's wrong and worries that Jeremy is losing interest in her.

What happened? First, Beverly delivered a fairly mild statement to Jeremy. Then Jeremy tormented himself with a whole host of anxiety-arousing words – *pig, totally, disgusted, never, impossible, certain,* and *unbearable.* Rather than ask Beverly for clarification, Jeremy let his mind overflow with powerful words that grossly distorted Beverly's original intention. His inner thoughts and the things he says to himself, which we call *self-talk,* far exceeded and indeed exaggerated the reality.

Worry words are words that provoke and increase anxiety. The worry words that you use when you think and talk to yourself easily inflame anxiety and are rarely supported by evidence or reality. Using them unwittingly becomes a bad habit. However, we have good news: Like any habit, the anxiety-arousing word habit can be broken.

Worry words come in four major categories. We'll go through each of them with you carefully.

- ✔ **Extremist:** Words that exaggerate or predict a catastrophe (*catastrophise*)

- ✔ **All-or-none:** Polar opposites with nothing in between

- ✔ **Judging, commanding, and labelling:** Harsh evaluations and name calling

- ✔ **Victim:** Words that underestimate your ability to cope

Extremist words

It's amazing how selecting certain words to describe events can make mountains out of molehills. Extremist words grossly magnify troubling situations. In doing so, they aggravate negative emotions.

Emily, pulling out of a tight parking space at the supermarket, recognises a neighbour coming out of the store and hoots to get her attention. As the sound of the horn dies away, Emily hears metal scraping metal. Her bumper dents a side panel of the latest-model people-carrier parked next to her. Emily slams on her brakes, yanks on the handbrake, and leaps out to inspect the damage. There's a four-inch long dent.

Using her mobile, she calls her husband, Ron, immediately. Hysterical, she cries, 'There's been a *horrible* accident. I *destroyed* the other car. I feel *awful;* I just *can't stand it.* You've got to come here right away.' Ron attempts to calm his wife and rushes to the scene from work. When he arrives, he's not surprised to find that the damage is far less extensive than his wife described. He's well aware of her habit of using extreme words, but that doesn't mean Emily isn't upset. She is. But neither she nor Ron realises how Emily's language adds fuel to the fire of her emotional response.

Most of Emily's problematic language falls under the category of extremist words. See the following list for examples of extremist words:

Abhorrent	Foul
Agonising	Ghastly
Appalling	Hopeless
Awful	Horrible
Catastrophic	Intolerable
Devastating	Terrible
Disastrous	Unbearable
Disgusting	Unimaginable
Dreadful	Unspeakable

Of course, reality can be horrible, appalling, and downright unspeakably, unimaginably awful. It would be hard to describe the Holocaust, 11 September 2001, famine, or the worldwide AIDS epidemic in milder terms. However, all too often, extremist words like these reshape reality. Think about how many times you or the people that you know use these words to describe events that, while certainly unpleasant, can hardly be described as utter calamities.

Life presents challenges for you to deal with: Loss, frustration, aggravation, and pain routinely drop in like unwelcome guests who annoy you considerably. You may try to banish them from your life, but your best efforts won't keep them from dropping in again, uninvited as usual. When they arrive, you have two choices. First, you can magnify and catastrophise and tell yourself how *horrible, awful, unbearable,* and *intolerable* they are. When you do that, you'll just intensify your anxiety and distress. Your other option is to think in more realistic terms. (See the 'Exorcising your extremist words' section, later in this chapter, for more about realistic options.)

All-or-none, black-or-white words

Pick up a black-and-white photograph. Any photo will do. Look carefully and you'll see many shades of grey that tend to dominate the picture. Most photos contain very little pure black or white at all. Calling a photo black and white oversimplifies matters and fails to capture the complexity and richness of the images. Just as calling a photograph black and white ignores much of the detail, describing an event in black-and-white terms ignores the full range of human experience. Like a photograph, very little in life is pure black or white.

Nevertheless, people easily slip into language that oversimplifies. Like extremist language, only using words that are opposites – black and white words – rather than the ones in between, intensifies negative feelings.

Thomas puts down his newspaper, unable to concentrate, and tells his wife that he'd better be off to work. 'I didn't sleep a wink last night. I've been *totally* freaked out about my sales target this month. I'll *never* reach it. There's *absolutely* no way. Sales *entirely* dried up with the slower economy, but the boss has *zero* tolerance for extenuating circumstances. I'm *certain* she's going to make an example of me. It would be *absolutely impossible* to find another job if she fires me.' If Thomas is at a loss for additional all-or-none words, he can borrow from the following list:

Absolute/absolutely	Invariably
All	Never
Always	No how
Ceaseless/ceaselessly	None
Complete/completely	No way
Constant/constantly	Perpetual/perpetually
Continuous/continuously	Total/totally
Entire/entirely	Without exception
Everyone/no-one	Zero
Forever	Zilch

Few things (other than death and taxes) occur with absolute certainty. You may recall pleading with your parents for a later curfew. We bet that you told them that *everyone* stays out later than you do. If so, you did it for good reason, hoping that the exaggeration would make a more powerful statement. Nevertheless, your parents probably saw through your ploy.

Everyone, and we really do mean everyone, exaggerates sometimes; our language has many words useful for just such purposes. Thomas exaggerates by declaring that he'll *never* reach his sales targets. Then his anxiety escalates. When Thomas states that he'll never reach his targets and that another job will be absolutely impossible to find, he concentrates on the negative rather than searching for positive solutions. But it doesn't have to be this way. For an all-or-none antidote, see the 'Disputing all-or-none words' section later in this chapter.

Judging words

Imagine that we had written the following, in all seriousness: You *must* read this book more carefully than you've been doing. Not only that, but you *should* have read more of it by now. And you *ought to* have taken the exercises more seriously. You're *just plain useless. Shame* on you! . . . (We're just kidding.)

What authors in the world would take their readers to task like that? None that we can think of. That sort of criticism is abusive. People react with dismay when they witness parents humiliating their children by calling them *stupid, useless,* or *rotten.* Many would view a teacher who calls his or her students *fools* and describes their best efforts as *awful, pathetic,* and *disgusting* as equally abusive. That kind of harsh judgement hardly inspires; in fact it crushes the will.

However, many people talk to themselves this way or even worse. Some hear a steady stream of critical commentary running through their minds. You may be your own worst critic. Many people take the critical voice that they heard in childhood and turn it on themselves, often magnifying the criticism in the process. (See Chapter 5 for more about critical voices in childhood.)

Steve, balancing his accounts, discovers that he neglected to enter a cheque a few days ago. Fretting that the cheque will bounce, Steve thinks, 'I *should* be more careful. It's *pathetic* that someone with a Master's degree can do something this *stupid.* I *ought* to know better. I'm such an *idiot.* I *disgust* myself. I *must never,* ever make this kind of mistake again.' By the time he finishes his self-abusive tirade, Steve feels more anxious and even a little depressed.

Judging words come in the following three varieties, and we show you examples in Table 7-1 in this chapter.

- ✔ **Judgements:** These are harsh judgements about yourself or what you do. For example, when you make an all-too-human mistake and call it an utter failure, you're judging your actions rather than merely describing them.

- ✔ **Commandments:** This category contains words that dictate absolute, unyielding rules about your behaviour or feelings. If you tell yourself that you *should* have taken or *must* take a particular action, you're listening to an internal drill sergeant. This zealous drill sergeant tolerates no deviation from a dogmatic code of conduct.

✔ **Labels:** Finally, self-degrading labels put the icing on the cake. Steve's accounting mistake, for example, leads to all three types of condemnations: He judges his error as *stupid,* he *shouldn't* have allowed it to happen, and he declares himself an *idiot.* It's no wonder that Steve feels anxious when he works on his accounts. Ironically, the increased anxiety makes further mistakes more likely.

Table 7-1	The Three Categories of Judging Words	
Judgements	*Commandments*	*Labels*
Bad	Have to	Fool
Despicable	Must	Imbecile
Failure	Ought	Idiot
Inadequate	Should	Twit
Pathetic	Or else!	A nothing
Stupid	Got to	A nobody
Undeserving	It's imperative	Pig
Feeble	It's vital	Greedy guts
Wrong		Wimp

Victim words

You may remember the story *The Little Engine That Could* by Watty Piper about the train that needed to climb a steep hill. The author of the book wisely chose not to have the engine say, 'I think I *can't;* I'll never do it; this hill's impossible.'

The world feels a much scarier place when you habitually think of yourself as a victim of circumstance. Certain words can serve as a flag for that kind of thinking, such as the list of victimising words that follows:

Can't	Overwhelmed
Defenceless	Powerless
Frail	Shattered
Helpless	Too much
Impossible	Vulnerable
Impotent	Worn out
Incapacitated	

Nadia, suffering from severe generalised anxiety, jumps whenever she hears loud noises. Married for 20 years to a husband who's been repeatedly unfaithful, Nadia doesn't consider leaving him, because she worries that she *can't* survive on her own. She feels *helpless* to deal with the demands of life on her own and believes that it would be *impossible* for her to handle working and caring for her two teenage kids. Even now, she feels *overwhelmed* by housework.

Victim words demoralise. They offer no hope. With no hope, there's little reason for positive action. When victims believe themselves to be defenceless, they feel vulnerable and afraid.

People who describe themselves as victims often don't feel compelled to even try to do much about whatever predicaments they face. Some people express sympathy for them, and others may offer to take care of them. Whether this constitutes much in the way of an advantage or compensation, we leave you to decide.

Tracking Your Worry Words

You probably don't realise how often you use worry words inside your head. Because worry words contribute to stress and anxiety, performing a check-up on your use of these words is a good idea. You can start by tuning in to your self-talk. Get a small notepad and carry it with you for a few days. Listen to what you say to yourself when you feel stressed or worried. Take a few minutes to record the internal chatter.

Now check your monologue for worry words. You may discover that you use a few worry words that we haven't listed and that some words may fit into more than one category. That's okay. Just look for the relevant themes. Underline them and then put them into these general categories (which we repeat from earlier in the chapter to save you time):

- ✔ **Extremist:** Words that exaggerate or predict a catastrophe (catastrophise)
- ✔ **All-or-none:** Polar opposites with nothing in between
- ✔ **Judging, commanding, and labelling:** Harsh evaluations and name calling
- ✔ **Victim:** Words that underestimate your ability to cope

Frank, a talented mechanic, works for a main dealer's garage. After his promotion to supervisor, he feels an enormous responsibility resting on his shoulders. Frank's punctuality, attention to detail, and perfectionism reflect his conscientious work ethic. Unfortunately, Frank's perfectionism goes too far. He worries about the quality of his team's work. He checks and rechecks everything. In order to feel like he's doing his job properly, he starts working 60 hours or more each week. His blood pressure starts to rise, and his doctor tells him that he needs to reduce his stress and anxiety.

So Frank picks up his copy of *Overcoming Anxiety For Dummies* and refers to Chapter 7 for help on tracking and trapping his worry words. This is what he writes:

> The workload is <u>dreadful</u>. It's <u>impossible</u> to keep up; I'm <u>overwhelmed</u>. But I <u>should</u> be able to do everything. I'm an <u>absolute failure</u> if I can't get all the work done. Because I'm the boss, I <u>must</u> be responsible for all the staff. If anyone doesn't do their job, I'm <u>totally</u> responsible. If someone else makes a mistake I <u>should</u> be on top of it. I <u>can't stand</u> the idea of a dissatisfied customer. When someone complains, it feels like a <u>calamity</u>. I feel like a <u>total failure</u> and a <u>fool</u> if I can't fix everything perfectly.

He finds that he has written worry words in all the main categories:

- ✔ **Extremist words:** *dreadful, calamity, can't stand it*
- ✔ **All-or-none words:** *totally, absolute*
- ✔ **Judging, commanding, and labelling words:** *total failure, fool, should, must*
- ✔ **Victim words:** *overwhelmed, impossible*

Frank is surprised to see how many worry words inhabit his thoughts. Yet he remains convinced that these words fit his reality. Frank needs to go a little further to overcome his anxiety.

Refuting and Replacing Your Worry Words

Ask yourself how you truly want to feel. Few people like feeling anxious, worried, and stressed. Who would choose those feelings? So perhaps you agree that you prefer to feel calm and serene rather than wound up. Set that as your goal.

A good way to start on your journey towards feeling better is to change your worry words. However, you aren't likely to stop using worry words just because we told you that they create anxiety. That's because you still may think that these words accurately describe yourself and/or your world. Many people go through life without questioning their self-talk, simply assuming that words equate with reality.

In order to refute the accuracy of your internal self-talk, consider a small change in philosophy. This shift entails questioning the idea that thoughts, language, and words automatically capture truth. Substitute that idea with a new one, using logic and evidence-gathering to structure your reality. At the same time, keep in mind that your goal is to experience greater calm.

Exorcising your extremist words

The vast majority of the time, when people use extremist words such as *intolerable, agonising, horrible, awful, hopeless,* and *ghastly,* they use them to describe everyday events. When you hear yourself using those words, subject them to a logical analysis.

For example, few events in life are really unbearable. After all, you managed to get through every single difficult time in your life up to now or you wouldn't be alive and reading this book. Many circumstances feel pretty awful, but somehow you deal with them. Life goes on.

When you think in extreme terms, using words such as *unbearable, intolerable, can't stand it, awful,* and *disastrous,* you lose hope. Your belief in your ability to manage and carry on diminishes. Consider whether your unpleasant experiences can be described more accurately in a different way; for example:

- ✔ Difficult but not unbearable
- ✔ Uncomfortable but not intolerable
- ✔ Disagreeable but not devastating
- ✔ Unpleasant but not unmanageable
- ✔ Distressing but not agonising

Recall Emily from the section 'Extremist words' earlier in the chapter. She dented a car in a car park accident and reacted with extreme distress, due in part to her thoughts based on extremist words. After she works on her exaggerated style, she learns to view minor problems for what they are – minor. For example, when her handbag is stolen from the changing room, she tells herself, 'Well, this sure is a hassle and a real pain. I don't like having to call the credit card companies to report that my cards have been stolen and apply for a copy of my driver's licence. But, at least I'll get the new-style photographic licence that I had to change to at some time. Plus I wasn't hurt and I can imagine far worse things.' Emily discovers she's far less upset when she thinks in these terms; she now can distinguish between a catastrophe and an inconvenience.

Remember your goal of feeling calmer. When you drop extreme language, the intensity of your emotions also drops. If you use words that describe things in moderate rather than extreme terms, this will soften your reactions. Less-extreme portrayals lead you to believe in your ability to cope. Humans have a surprising reservoir of resilience. You cultivate your capacity for problem solving and survival when you have hope.

Disputing all-or-none words

People use all-or-none words, such as *never, always, absolute, forever, unceasing,* and *constant,* because they're quick, easy, and they add emotional punch. But these terms have insidious downsides: They push your thinking to extremes, and your emotions tag along for the ride. Furthermore, all-or-none words detract from coping and problem solving.

Rarely does careful gathering of evidence support the use of all-or-none words. Many people use all-or-none words to predict the future or to describe the past. But look carefully and you'll see that people often talk about the past in the present tense; for example, 'You *always* criticise me' or 'I *never* get promoted.' This then states, in black and white terms, that this is the reality of the past, the present, and by implication the future as well. You are saying that that's what happened to you in the past and it's happening now, and you are predicting that it will always happen in the future – it's just the way it is! Whether you're talking to yourself or someone else, these words hardly facilitate calmness, nor do they describe what really happened or what's likely to happen in the future. So try to stay in the present and also to drop those all-or-none words.

Table 7-2 illustrates the switch between all-or-none words and calm, evidence-gathering words that keep you *in the present without exaggeration.*

Table 7-2	Switching to the Present
All or None	*In the Present without Exaggeration*
I *never* get promoted.	At this moment, I don't know whether I'll be promoted. However, I'll do everything that I can to see to it that I am.
You *always* criticise me.	Right now, you are criticising me, and that's making me unhappy.
I always panic when I'm in a crowd.	Right now, I can't know for certain whether I'll panic the next time I'm in a crowd. I may panic, and I may not. If I do, it's not the worst thing in the world, and I won't die from it.

Remember Thomas from the earlier section of this chapter on all-or-none, black-or-white words? Thomas thought he'd never make his sales target and that he'd probably be fired. After being sacked, he assumed he would never find another job. After reading *Overcoming Anxiety For Dummies,* Thomas realises his own words have hurt him. He changes his words to reflect shades of grey. A few months later, he actually fails to reach his sales quota. Rather than catastrophise, he thinks, 'Okay, this wasn't a great month. I wasn't the only one to miss the target, and it's very unlikely I'll be fired. If I do get fired, my sales record will probably land me another job. I'm going to stop worrying and focus on doing my best to achieve next month's target.'

Thomas moves from despair to reasonable optimism. His stress goes down and his sales increase. You can do the same for yourself, no matter what your problem.

Judging the judging words

Words that judge, command, or label, such as *should, must, failure, fool, undeserving,* and *twit,* inflict unnecessary pain and shame on their recipients. You may hear these words from others or from your own critic within.

Labels and judgements describe a person as a whole, but people usually use them to describe a specific action. For example, if you make a mistake, you may say to yourself, 'I can't believe that I could be such an *idiot!*' If you say this, you make a global evaluation of your entire being based on a single action. Is that useful? Clearly it's not accurate, and most importantly, the judgement doesn't lead you to feel calm or serene or to believe that you can do anything to prevent such mistakes in the future. Being the idiot you are, you'll just keep repeating the same mistakes plus new ones – won't you? – because that's just what fools like you do; they never learn from their mistakes. We trust you can see how extremely unhelpful this line of thought is and the dangerous places to which it can lead. Carry on like this long enough and you risk convincing yourself it is true. As well as feeling more anxious, you could also start feeling depressed.

Like the other types of worry words, commandments don't inspire motivation and seldom improve performance. Yet people use these words for those very purposes. They think that saying I *must* or I *should* will help them, but it's more likely that those words will cause them to feel guilty or anxious. Self-scolding merely increases guilt and anxiety, and guilt and anxiety inevitably decrease both motivation and performance.

Try replacing your judging, commanding, and labelling words with more reasonable, accurate, and supportable alternatives:

 ✔ **Judging:** I got pathetic results for my end-of-term exams. I must be stupid.

   Reasonable alternative: It wasn't the result that I wanted, but I can study more and do better next term. Given how little work I actually did, the results were pretty reasonable.

 ✔ **Commanding:** I must have a happy marriage. I should have what it takes to keep it happy, so it must be all my fault if problems arise.

   Reasonable alternative: Much as I'd like to have a happy marriage, I was okay before I met my wife, and I can learn to be okay again if I have to. Being happily married is just my strong preference, and I don't have complete control over the outcome; it does take two, after all.

In the earlier section 'Judging words', Steve made an error in his accounts. He promptly condemned himself by calling himself a fool and telling himself he should never make an error like that again. After Steve tackles this bad habit, he changes his views. Like most people, Steve makes another mistake in his cheque book three months later. This time he realises the world will not end and that he is not stupid. He stops and reflects. Reflection allows him to see that most of his mistakes happen when he tries to do two or three tasks at once. He decides to slow down a little. Using less harsh judgements allows Steve to learn from his mistakes rather than berate himself.

Vanquishing victim words

Victim words, such as *powerless, helpless, vulnerable, overwhelmed,* and *defenceless,* put you in a deep hole and fill you with a sense of vulnerability and fear. They make you feel as though finding a way out is impossible and that hope remains out of reach. Yet, as with other worry words, only rarely do they convey unmitigated truth. It is worth remembering the old adage that when you find yourself in a hole, it's best to stop digging.

Victim words can become what are known as self-fulfilling prophecies. If you *think* that a goal is impossible, you're not likely to achieve it, and there will be little point in attempting it at all. If you *think* that you're powerless, you won't draw upon your coping resources. Instead, you're likely to remain stuck in your adversity. As an alternative, consider the logic of your victim words. Is there anything at all that you can do to remedy or at least improve your problem?

Gather evidence for refuting victim words that appear in your self-talk. Ask yourself whether you've ever managed to cope with a similar situation before. Think about a friend, an acquaintance, or anyone at all who has successfully dealt with a burden like yours.

A survivor's story

A large window shattered and sliced Karen Smyers' hamstring, which required surgery. That was in 1997. In 1998, an articulated lorry hit Karen from behind while she was riding her bike, leaving her with six broken ribs and a badly damaged shoulder. In 1999, she broke her collarbone and found out that she had thyroid cancer. The year after the surgery to remove her thyroid gland, doctors discovered cancerous lymph nodes in her neck. Karen considers herself lucky. In October 2001, at age 40, she won a triathlon in Austin, Texas. Karen focused on her goals and her family in spite of adversities that many would consider overwhelming.

After you consider the logic and the evidence, ask whether victim words make you feel better, calmer, or less anxious. If not, replace those words with new ones; for example:

✔ **Victim:** I have a fatal disease, and I'm totally powerless to do anything about it.

Reasonable alternative: I have a disease that's indeed often fatal. However, I can explore every avenue from clinical trials to alternative treatments. If that doesn't work, I can still find meaning with the rest of my life.

✔ **Victim:** I feel overwhelmed by debt. I feel helpless and have no options other than declaring bankruptcy.

Reasonable alternative: I do have a considerable debt. However, I can go to a debt adviser who specialises in renegotiating interest rates and payments. I may also be able to get a second part-time job and chip away at the bills. If ultimately I do have to declare bankruptcy, I can slowly rebuild my credit.

Recall Nadia from the earlier section 'Victim words'. She remains married to a husband who cheats on her repeatedly. Nadia feels there's no way out, because she can never be okay on her own. After considerable therapy, Nadia no longer views herself as a victim. She stands up to her husband, insists they seek marital therapy, and tells him that if he continues to cheat on her, she will leave him. She knows that she can survive on her own. Stunned by her new-found assertiveness, her husband finds her more attractive. He agrees to marital therapy and recommits to the marriage.

Part III
Acting Against Anxiety

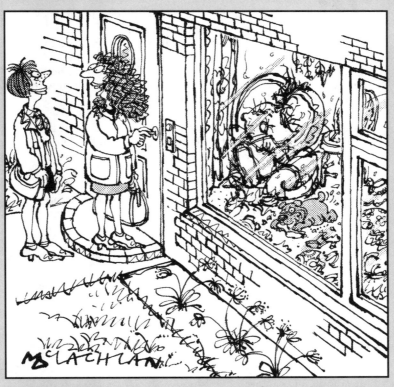

'A friend told me that a pet helps with anxiety so today I bought myself a puppy.'

In this part . . .

We show you that changing what you're doing is another powerful way to attack anxiety. We provide you with a set of tools for challenging your fears by facing them head-on. Don't worry; we help you do this gradually, one step at a time. This part helps you to figure out what's important to you; then you can find out how to streamline your life in ways that fit your goals.

You'll also see how exercise can reduce your anxiety. If you struggled in the past with getting yourself to exercise, we help you see why and what you can do to find the motivation.

Finally, after all that activity, you're going to need some sleep. That's one reason why we show you various ways of improving your sleep.

Chapter 8

Facing Fear One Step at a Time

Sharon sets out to master riding a bike without training wheels. Grandpa holds the bike steady and jogs along beside her. Sharon beams with pride. She is doing fine, but the second that Grandpa tells her that she's doing great without his help, Sharon gets scared, realising that she's on her own. Before Grandpa can grab on, Sharon and the bike crash into a heap. Both knees bloody, Sharon cries in real pain.

Grandpa comforts Sharon and tells her, 'There's an old saying: When you fall off a horse, get right back on. So let's get you cleaned up and put on some plasters; then we'll give it another try.'

Good advice, but Sharon finds herself paralysed with fear, unable to face having another go. Nevertheless, after a few days, she manages to try again, and this time all goes according to plan. In fact, she so enjoys cycling she eventually competes in the Women's Tour de France. Not everyone who gets hurt in life can do that.

When life hands you lemons, make lemonade. But is this advice really as easy to put into action as it seems? Is turning a situation around for the better after a series of hurts, or even bouncing back after one difficulty, a realistic self-expectation?

This chapter explains how you can get back in the saddle and overcome your fears in manageable steps. We discuss how to face fears in your imagination. That prepares you for the next step of tackling your fears by facing them head on, but in small steps. This chapter also provides a recipe called *exposure* for overcoming your personal anxiety problems.

Exposure: Coming to Grips with Your Fears

No single strategy discussed in this book works more effectively in the fight against anxiety than exposure. Simply put, exposure involves putting yourself in direct contact with whatever it is that makes you anxious. Well now, that may just sound a little ridiculous to you.

After all, it probably makes you feel pretty anxious to even think about staring your fears in the face. We understand that reaction, but please realise that if you're terrified of heights, exposure doesn't ask you to go on the London Eye tomorrow or climb Ben Nevis. Or if you worry about having a panic attack in crowds, you don't have to sit in the stands of the new Wembley Stadium as your first step.

If you find yourself procrastinating with the recommendations in this chapter, read Chapter 3 on how to build motivation and overcome obstacles to change. If you still find these ideas difficult to consider, you may want to consult a professional for help.

Graded exposure – taking one step at a time

Exposure involves a systematic, gradual set of steps that you can tackle one at a time. You don't move from the first step until you master it. Then, when you're comfortable with the first one, you move to the second. While it's true that each new step brings on anxiety, you'll find it's not an overwhelming amount.

Don't try exposure if your anxiety is severe. You'll need professional guidance. If any step raises your anxiety to an extreme level, stop any further self-help attempts unless you get professional help as well. Also, don't attempt exposure if you're in the midst of a crisis or have a current problem with alcohol or substance abuse.

Getting ready

Before you do anything else, we suggest that you practise relaxing. Consider reading Chapters 12 and 13 for a thorough review of how to do this. But for now, you can use a couple of simple, quick methods.

Why practise relaxing? Exposure makes you anxious. No way around that. Working out how to relax can help you feel more confident about dealing with that anxiety. Relaxation can help keep the inevitable anxiety within tolerable limits.

First, we suggest a breathing strategy:

1. **Inhale slowly, deeply, and fully through your nose.**

2. **Hold your breath for a slow count of six.**

3. **Slowly breathe out through your mouth to a count of eight, while making a slight hissing or sighing sound as you do. That sound can be ever so soft.**

4. **Repeat this type of breath ten times.**

Try practising this type of breathing several times a day. See how it makes you feel. If it doesn't help you feel calmer, stop doing it. Instead, try our next suggestion, which tightens and loosens muscle groups, an abbreviation of the method discussed in Chapter 12.

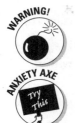

If you have any physical problems, such as lower back pain, recent injury, surgery, muscle spasms, or severe arthritic conditions, don't use the technique that follows. If you think that you can, do so gently and be sure to avoid tensing up to the point of pain, even if you're in good condition.

1. **Find a comfortable place to sit or lie down.**

2. **Loosen any tight clothing.**

3. **Flex your feet and point your toes up towards your knees.**

4. **Clamp your legs together.**

5. **Tighten all the muscles in your feet, legs, and buttocks.**

6. **Hold the tension for a count of eight.**

7. **Now release the tension all at once.**

8. **Allow relaxation to slowly come in and replace the tension.**

9. **Notice the relaxed feeling for a few moments.**

10. **Next, squeeze your fists, bring your hands up to your shoulders, pull in your stomach, and pull your shoulder blades back as though you're trying to make them touch. Tighten all the muscles between your waist and your neck. Hold for eight seconds.**

11. **Release the tension, allow relaxation to replace the tension, and notice the relaxed feeling.**

12. **Finally, tense your neck and facial muscles. Scrunch your face into a tight ball.**

13. **Hold the tension for eight seconds.**

14. **Release the tension and relax. Be aware of the relaxation as it slowly replaces the tension.**

15. **Stay with the new, relaxed feelings for a few minutes.**

16. **If you still feel tense, repeat the procedure one more time.**

Most people find that one or both of the breathing or the muscle-tensing exercise techniques relax them, even if only a little. If by any chance these techniques fail to relax you or even make you more anxious, Chapters 12 and 13 may give you more ideas. Work through those chapters carefully.

However, even if no relaxation technique works for you, it doesn't mean that exposure won't be effective. Exposure can work on its own. Without relaxation, you simply need to proceed more slowly and carefully.

Building blocks

Breaking down the exposure process into manageable steps is important. To start the process:

1. **Pick one and only one of your worries – perhaps there's one within the following list of examples:**

   • Enclosed spaces

   • Financial ruin

   • Flying

   • Having a panic attack (a fear of a fear)

   • People

2. **Think about every conceivable aspect of your fear or worry.**

   What triggers your fear? Include all the activities surrounding your fear. For example, if you're afraid of flying, perhaps you fear driving to the airport or packing your luggage. Or if you're afraid of dogs, you avoid walking near them, and you probably don't visit people who have dogs in their homes. Whenever the fear occurs, take some notes on it. Think about all the anticipated and feared outcomes. Include all the details, such as other people's reactions and the setting.

Gail's story is a good illustration of how to break down the exposure process into manageable steps:

Gail, a 32-year-old sales representative for a pharmaceutical company, receives a promotion, putting her in charge of the North American Division. This means a large increase in salary and plenty of air travel. During her interview, Gail doesn't mention her intense fear of flying, somehow hoping that it will just go away. In three weeks she faces her first flight, and her distress prompts her to seek help.

Luckily for her, Gail picks up a copy of *Overcoming Anxiety For Dummies*. She reads about exposure and concludes that it's the best approach for her problem. To see how Gail completes the first task of describing her fear and all its components, see Table 8-1.

Table 8-1	What I'm Afraid Of
Question	*Answer*
How does my anxiety begin?	The very thought of flying makes me anxious. Even driving on the road that leads to the airport gets me worked up.
What activities does my fear include?	First, I'd have to book a ticket – that would be difficult. Then I'd have to pack my luggage, drive to the airport, go through security, spend some time in the departure lounge, hear my flight called, and board the plane. Then I'd take a seat and go through take-off. Finally, I'd endure the flight.
What outcomes do I anticipate?	I fear that I'll go crazy, throw up on the passengers next to me, or start screaming, and the cabin crew will have to restrain me. Of course, the plane may crash, and I'd die or sustain horrible burns and pain, unable to get out of the plane. I may even crash and then be eaten alive by alligators.

You can see that Gail's fear of flying involves of a number of activities, from making a reservation to getting off the plane. Her anticipated outcomes include a range of distinctly unpleasant possibilities.

Using the Table 8-1 question-and-answer format, you can describe what you're afraid of. Use your imagination. Don't let embarrassment keep you from including the deepest, darkest aspects of your fears, even though they may sound silly to someone else.

Now, you're ready to take your fear apart and stack your building blocks. Use your blocks to construct a tower of fear (see Figure 8-1). Make a list of each aspect of your fear. Then rate each one on a scale of 0 to 100. Zero represents the total absence of fear, and 100 indicates a fear that's unimaginably intense and totally debilitating. Then stack your blocks with the lowest-ranked block at the bottom and the highest ranked one at the top. This constitutes your exposure hierarchy.

Figure 8-1 shows how Gail stacked the blocks for her fear of flying.

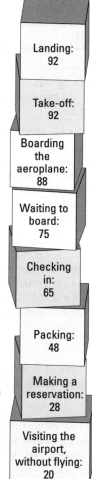

Figure 8-1:
How Gail ranks her fears about flying.

Landing: 92

Take-off: 92

Boarding the aeroplane: 88

Waiting to board: 75

Checking in: 65

Packing: 48

Making a reservation: 28

Visiting the airport, without flying: 20

Gail's tower contains only eight building blocks. You may want to break the task down into 15 or 20 steps. For example, Gail's steps jump from packing to checking in. She can add several steps in between, such as driving to the airport and parking in the airport car park.

For a phobia like Gail's, the building blocks represent tasks that all directly lead to her ultimate fear. But some people have different types of anxiety. For example, someone with generalised anxiety disorder (GAD; see Chapter 2), may have a variety of fears – a fear of rejection, fear of getting hurt, and worry about financial calamity. The most effective tower of fear chooses one of those fears and includes everything relevant to that fear.

So, now you have your tower of fear. What do you do next? Choose between the two kinds of exposure – the kind that occurs in your imagination and the exposure that occurs in real life.

Do remember, if you don't go looking for your fear, chances are it comes looking for you.

Imagining the worst

Many times, the best way to begin exposure is in your imagination. That's because imagining your fears usually elicits less anxiety than actually confronting them directly. In addition, you can use your imagination when it would be impossible to replicate your real fear. For example, if you fear getting a disease, such as hepatitis C, actually exposing yourself to the virus wouldn't be a good idea.

You may think that viewing your fears through your mind's eye wouldn't make you anxious. However, most people find that when they picture their fears in rich detail, their bodies react. As they gradually master their fears in their minds, generally the fears reduce when confronting the real-life version.

Imaginary exposure follows just a few basic steps:

1. If you think it would make you more comfortable, use one of the brief relaxation strategies described in the 'Getting ready' section, earlier in this chapter, before you start.

2. Choose the lowest building block from your tower of fear.

3. Picture yourself as if you are actually confronting your fear. Gail's first block was visiting the airport without any intention of flying.

4. Imagine as many details about your fear building block as you can – include the sights, sounds, smells, and anything that brings your imaginary experience to life. If you have difficulty picturing the experience, see Chapter 13 for ideas on how to sharpen your mind's eye.

5. When you have a good picture in your mind that gives you an idea of what being exposed to your fear would be like, rate your anxiety on a scale of 0 to 100, where 0 is equivalent to no anxiety at all, and 100 to the most terror you could ever imagine experiencing.

6. Keeping the picture in your mind, practise your relaxation, until you feel your anxiety drop significantly. Waiting until your rating decreases by around half or more is best. It will come down that much as long as you stay with the imaginary exposure long enough. For example, if you experience anxiety at a level 60, keep thinking about the exposure image until your anxiety drops to around 30.

7. Finish the session with a further brief relaxation technique – one of those described in the 'Getting ready' section earlier in this chapter.

8. If the imaginary experience wasn't particularly scary, you may want to choose the next building block, a step up in your tower of fear, and perhaps another one after that. Continue daily practice. Always start with the last building block that you completed successfully (in other words, one for which your anxiety level dropped by half or more).

Facing your fears (gulp)

Although we usually recommend starting exposure in your imagination, the most effective type of exposure happens in real life. The strategy works in much the same way as imaginary exposure; you break your fears down into small steps and stack them into a tower of fear from the least problematic to the most intensely feared. Now, it's time to face your fears head on. Gulp.

1. **Start with a brief relaxation procedure, such as the one of those described earlier in this chapter.**

2. **Select a fear or a group of worries with a similar theme, such as fear of rejection or risk of personal injury.**

3. **Next, break the fear into a number of sequential steps, each step being slightly more difficult than the prior step.**

4. **Finally, take one step at a time.** If your anxiety starts to rise to an unmanageable level, try using one of the brief relaxation techniques. Keep working on each step until your anxiety drops, generally by at least half.

See the following hints to help you get through the exposure process:

- ✔ Get help from your partner or a friend, but only if that person is someone you really trust. This person can give you encouragement and support.

- ✔ If you must, take a small step back. Don't make a complete retreat unless you absolutely feel out of control.

- Your mind will tell you, 'Stop! You can't do this. It won't work anyway.' Don't listen to this chatter. Simply study your body's reactions and realise that they will not harm you.

- Find a way to reward yourself for each successful step that you take. Perhaps indulge in some desired purchase or treat yourself in some other way.

- Use a little positive self-talk to help quell rising anxiety, if you need to. See Chapter 5 for ideas.

- Understand that at times you will feel uncomfortable. View that discomfort as progress; it is part of how you overcome your fears.

- Practise, practise, and practise.

- Don't forget to practise a brief relaxation procedure before and during the exposure.

- Remember to stay with each step until your anxiety drops. Realise that your body can't maintain anxiety forever. It will calm down if you give it sufficient time.

- Expect exposure to take time. Go at a reasonable pace. Keep moving forwards, but remember that you don't have to conquer your fear in a few days. Even with daily practice, self-exposure can take a number of months.

Remember to choose realistic goals. For example, let's say you're afraid of spiders, so much so that you can't enter a room without an exhaustive search for hidden horrors. You don't have to get to the point where you let tarantulas crawl up and down your arms. Let yourself feel satisfied with the ability to enter rooms without unnecessary checking. And if you do see a spider, either to be able to ignore it until it goes away or use a glass and a piece of cardboard to pick it up and deposit it outside.

Finally, try to avoid using crutches during exposure. People use crutches, such as alcohol and drugs, to avoid fully exposing themselves to the steps in their towers of fear. Some of the popular crutches that people use include the following:

- Drinking – either alcohol or water. Some people say they won't go anywhere unless they take a bottle of water that they can sip if they start to feel anxious. So while drinking water is a great idea generally, do be careful that you aren't using it as a crutch and telling yourself that you can't manage without it.

- Taking tranquilisers, especially the benzodiazepines discussed in Chapter 15.

- Distracting yourself with rituals, song lyrics, or chants.

- Holding on to something to keep from falling or fainting.

If you absolutely feel the need to use one of these crutches, use it as little as you can. Sometimes, a reasonable in-between step is to use lyrics or chants at first and then repeat that step in your tower of fear without the chants.

In your later steps, it would be good to even drop relaxation, as a way to completely master your fear. This will give you the confidence that even at times when you aren't completely relaxed, you can still manage your anxiety and not be overwhelmed by it.

Conquering Your Fears

Confronting your fears directly is one of the most powerful ways of overcoming them. The exposure plan can look different, depending on the particular type of anxiety that you have. This section lays out sample plans for six types of anxiety. You'll no doubt need to individualise these for dealing with your problem. However, they should help you to get started.

You may want to review the detailed descriptions of the seven major types of anxiety in Chapter 2. We are omitting one of them: post-traumatic stress disorder. That's because, for the most part, people with this disorder should seek professional advice. The list that follows offers a brief synopsis of each anxiety category for which we suggest the use of real-life exposure:

- **Generalised anxiety disorder (GAD):** A chronic, long-lasting state of tension and worry.

- **Social phobia:** A fear of rejection, humiliation, or negative judgement from others.

- **Specific phobia:** An exaggerated, intense fear of some specific object, such as a needle; an animal, such as a spider; or a situation, such as being high off the ground – otherwise known as acrophobia, a fear of heights.

- **Panic disorder:** A fear of experiencing repeated panic attacks in which you feel a variety of physical symptoms, such as light-headedness, racing heartbeat, or nausea. You may also fear losing control, dying, or going crazy.

- **Agoraphobia:** This problem often, but not always, accompanies panic disorder. You worry about leaving home, feeling trapped, or feeling unable to get help if you should need it.

- **Obsessive-compulsive disorder:** Repetitive, unwanted thoughts jump into your mind and disturb you. This disorder can also involve various actions that you perform repeatedly as a way to prevent something bad from happening. Frequently, these actions don't make much sense, but they make you feel better, safer, and less anxious.

Waging war on worry: GAD

People with generalised anxiety disorder (GAD) worry about nearly everything. As a result of that worry, they usually end up avoiding a variety of opportunities plus the tasks of everyday life. These worries can rob people of pleasure and enjoyment.

Maureen's friends call her a real worrier and her children call her the prison warder. Maureen frets constantly, but her biggest worry is the safety of her 15-year-old twin boys. Unfortunately, Maureen's worry causes her to restrict her sons' activities far more than most parents do.

She drives them to and from school, much to their embarrassment, and won't hear of them taking public transport, even though there's a good bus service from where they live to the school, which all the other local pupils take. Maureen also acts as family taxi driver and prefers to have the boys' new friends visit the home, which enables her to vet all friends and keep tabs on the boys' activities.

The boys have to get Maureen's permission to attend any after-school activities, as this involves a change in routine for Maureen, and she interrogates them about everything they do at school and about all their friends.

As her sons get older, they rebel. Squabbles and fights dominate dinner, but the biggest bone of contention revolves around their desire to get mopeds for their 16th birthdays. It's not just the cost, of course, which worries Maureen. She frets continuously about the safety of her sons on one of those machines.

Maureen finds she's getting increasingly anxious and irritable with her children and even a bit depressed with the constant arguments. She goes to her GP for help. The GP suggests Maureen sees the practice counsellor for sessions, and she agrees.

During discussions with the counsellor, the issue of Maureen's sons' need for greater independence emerges. The counsellor helps Maureen to see that this is a very normal stage for parents to go through, when they need to let go and allow their children to learn the skills that will make them effective adults. The counsellor encourages Maureen to talk to friends and other parents with children of a similar age and find out about what level of independence they see as acceptable. She finds out that most parents allow their children to travel on the buses freely. Parents are divided on the subject of personal transport at 16, but those considering it point out that when you buy a new moped, you can often also get initial safety training with the bike.

Maureen constructs her tower of fear, stacking the blocks from the least fearful to the most terrifying (see Figure 8-2). She rates the anxiety that each block causes her on a scale from 0 to 100. Then she rates her anxiety again with repeated exposures. She doesn't go to the next step until her anxiety comes down by about a half.

Maureen's entire tower of fear actually consists of 20 blocks, but we've only shown the last five. Maureen tries to make sure that each step is within five to ten anxiety points of the previous one.

If you have GAD, pick one of your various worries. Then construct your personal tower of fear.

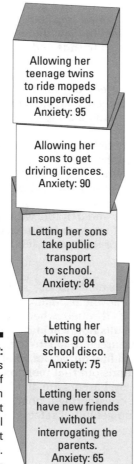

Allowing her teenage twins to ride mopeds unsupervised.
Anxiety: 95

Allowing her sons to get driving licences.
Anxiety: 90

Letting her sons take public transport to school.
Anxiety: 84

Letting her twins go to a school disco.
Anxiety: 75

Letting her sons have new friends without interrogating the parents.
Anxiety: 65

Figure 8-2:
Maureen's tower of fear, with the most fearful situations at the top.

Construct your tower with enough blocks so that the steps are small. If you find one step insurmountable, try coming up with an in-between step. If you can't do that, try doing the next step through repeated imaginary exposure before tackling it in real life.

Fighting phobias – specific and social

You fight both specific and social phobias in pretty much the same way. Take the feared situation, object, or animal and approach it in graded steps. Again, you construct a tower of fear out of steps or building blocks.

Eric's story is a good example of how the tower of fear can help someone with a specific phobia – a fear of heights.

Eric meets Diane through an online singles chat room. They e-mail back and forth for several weeks. Finally, they decide to meet for coffee. Several hours pass in what seem like minutes to both of them, and Eric offers to walk Diane home.

Leaving the bistro, Eric holds the door open for Diane, and Diane's body brushes against him. Their eyes meet and Eric almost kisses her right there in the doorway. As they walk towards her block of flats, she asks, 'Do you believe in love at first sight?' Eric doesn't hesitate: 'Yes', he answers, wrapping her in his arms. The kiss is so intense that Eric thinks he may collapse on the spot.

'I've never done this before on a first date, but I think I'd like you to come up to my place.' Diane strokes his arm. 'I have a wonderful view of the entire city from my penthouse.'

Eric looks up at the 15-storey building. His desire evaporates. 'Ah, well, I've got to pick up my sister, I mean go home to set the video', he stammers. Diane, obviously hurt and surprised, snaps, 'Fine. I've really got to wash my hair.'

Eric decides to fight his phobia. He constructs a tower of fear out of building blocks that start with what he wants to achieve and go all the way to the least fearful step:

- ✔ Visiting Diane in her penthouse and looking out from the balcony. Anxiety: 95

- ✔ Visiting Diane in her penthouse but not going out onto the balcony. Instead, looking out at the city from inside her living room. Anxiety: 82

- ✔ Going up in a hotel lift on my own to the tenth floor and looking out. Anxiety: 80

- ✔ Taking the glass hotel lift to the tenth floor with Diane and looking out. Anxiety: 75

 ✔ Imagining visiting Diane in her penthouse and going out onto the balcony, as well as peering down. Anxiety: 68

 ✔ Walking up three flights of stairs and peering down. Anxiety: 62

 ✔ Walking across a pedestrian bridge that has a chain-link fence around it. Anxiety: 55

 ✔ Imagining visiting Diane in her penthouse apartment without going onto the balcony. Anxiety: 53

 ✔ Calling Diane and telling her about my phobia, and hopefully getting her understanding and support. Anxiety: 48

Confessing his problem to Diane is a building block that may appear unrelated to Eric's fear. However, not admitting to his fear is avoidance, which only fuels fear. Including any building block that's connected to your fear is good.

Eric also included building blocks in his tower that require him to use his imagination to face his fear. It's fine to do that. Sometimes, an imaginary building block can help you take the next behavioural step.

Imagining the real-life steps before actually doing them doesn't hurt.

Pushing through panic and agoraphobia

Even if you only have panic disorder without agoraphobia, you can approach it in much the same way as you do agoraphobia. That's because your panic attacks are likely to have predictable triggers. Those triggers can form the basis for your tower of fear.

Felicity, for example, experiences her first panic attack shortly after the birth of her baby. Always somewhat shy, she begins to worry about something happening to herself when she takes the baby out. She fears that she may faint or lose control, and the baby would be vulnerable to harm.

Her panic attacks start with a feeling of nervousness and sweaty palms, and then progress to shallow, rapid breathing, a racing heartbeat, light-headedness, and a sense of dread and doom. Venturing away from the house triggers her attacks, and the more crowded the destination, the more likely that she'll experience panic. By six months after her first attack, she rarely leaves the house without her husband.

One day, Felicity's baby girl has a high temperature and a serious fever, and she needs to take her to A&E. Panic overtakes her; she frantically calls her husband, but he's out on a business call. Desperate, she calls 999 to send an ambulance, knowing all the while that it would be faster to drive to the nearby hospital herself.

Felicity knows that she must do something about her panic disorder and its companion, agoraphobia. She constructs a tower of fear out of a set of building blocks, starting with the least problematic and then going on to the top, most difficult goal:

- ✔ Taking the baby by myself to the shopping centre on Saturday afternoon, when it's most crowded. Anxiety: 98

- ✔ Taking the baby to the local shops during the day, when they're only moderately crowded. Anxiety: 92

- ✔ Going without the baby or my husband to the shopping centre when it's crowded. Anxiety: 88

- ✔ Going with the baby to the local shop when it first opens, when hardly anyone is there. Anxiety: 86

- ✔ Going by myself to the local shop when it's only moderately crowded. Anxiety: 84

- ✔ Taking the baby to the doctor by myself. Anxiety: 80

- ✔ Taking the baby on three errands in one day. Anxiety: 74

- ✔ Taking the baby to the bank when it's crowded. Anxiety: 65

- ✔ Taking the baby in the car to my mother's house, five miles away, for the afternoon. Anxiety: 30

- ✔ Walking the baby around the block. Anxiety: 25

Notice that Felicity's tower of fear contains quite a few steps between 80 and her top item of 98. That's because she needs to make each step very gradual in order to have the courage to proceed. She could have made the steps even smaller if necessary.

You can break your tower of fear down into as many small steps as you need so you do not feel overwhelmed by taking any single step.

One final type of exposure with panic attacks involves experiencing the sensations of the attacks themselves. How do you do that? You intentionally bring them on through carrying out for a short while any of the strategies that follow:

- ✔ **Running on the spot, or up and down stairs:** This accelerates your heartbeat, just as it would during many panic attacks.

- ✔ **Spinning yourself around until you feel dizzy:** Panic attacks often include sensations of dizziness and light-headedness.

- ✔ **Breathing through a small cocktail straw:** This strategy induces sensations of not getting enough air, which also mimics panic.

> ✔ **Putting your head between your knees and then standing up suddenly:** You may feel light-headed or dizzy.
>
> ✔ **Taking rapid, shallow breaths for three minutes:** This can make you may feel light-headed, dizzy, or a bit unreal.

After you have experienced these physical sensations on many occasions, you discover that they don't harm you. You won't go crazy, have a heart attack, or lose control. Frequent, prolonged exposure begins to convince you that sensations are just sensations, and that they don't lead to catastrophic consequences.

Don't bring on these physical sensations if you have a serious heart condition or any other physical problem that may be exacerbated by the exercise. For example, if you have asthma or a back injury, some of these strategies would be ill-advised. Check with your doctor if you have any questions or concerns.

Overcoming Obsessive-Compulsive Disorder

Obsessive-compulsive disorder (OCD) sometimes overwhelms and dominates a person's life, and commonly requires help from a professional with experience treating this disorder. Only attempt the strategies that we describe in this section on your own if your problems with OCD are relatively mild. Even then, you may want to enlist a friend or partner to help you.

Chapter 2 discusses this disorder, which often starts with obsessive, unwanted thoughts that create anxiety. People with this problem then try to relieve the anxiety caused by their thoughts by performing one of a number of compulsive acts. Unfortunately, it seems that the relief obtained from the compulsive acts only fuels the vicious cycle.

Therefore, for OCD, exposure is only the first step. Then you must do something even harder, which is to stop carrying out the compulsive, anxiety-relieving actions. This strategy has a rather obvious name, *exposure and response prevention*.

But let's start with the first step of exposure. Because OCD has an obsessional component – in other words, feared thoughts, images, and impulses – exposure often starts with imaginary exposure, as described in the 'Imagining the worst' section earlier in this chapter. Imaginary exposure may be the only strategy that you can use if your obsessions couldn't or shouldn't be acted out in real life, such as in the following examples:

> ✔ Thoughts that tell you to violate your personal religious beliefs
>
> ✔ Repetitive thoughts of harm coming to a family member or loved one
>
> ✔ Frequent worries about burning alive in a home fire
>
> ✔ Unwanted thoughts about getting cancer or some other dreaded disease

Now do the following:

1. **List your distressing thoughts and images and then rate each one for the amount of distress it causes.**

2. **Next, select the thought that causes the least upset and dwell on the thought over and over, until your distress abates by at least half.**

   Sometimes, listening over and over to a tape-recorded description of your obsession is useful.

3. **Then proceed to the next item on your list that causes a little more discomfort and keep working your way up the list.**

This approach is quite the opposite of what people with OCD usually do with their unwanted obsessions. Normally, they try to sweep the haunting thoughts out of their minds the moment that they appear, but that only succeeds ever so briefly, and it maintains the cycle.

Give imaginary exposure enough time and keep the thoughts and images in your head long enough for your anxiety to reduce by at least half before moving on to the next item.

If you also suffer from compulsive acts, or avoidance due to obsessive thoughts, it's now time for the more difficult, second step of real-life, or in–vivo, exposure and response prevention. Again, make a hierarchy of feared events and situations that you typically avoid – the tower of fear – and then proceed to put yourself into each of those situations, but without performing the compulsive act.

For example, if you fear contamination from dirt and grime, go to a beach, play in the sand, and build sandcastles, or go out in the garden, plant flowers, and keep yourself from washing your hands. Remain in the situation until your distress drops by half. If it doesn't drop that much, stay at least an hour and a half and try not to quit until a minimum of a third of your distress goes away. Don't proceed to the next item until you conquer the one that you're working on.

Although using relaxation procedures with initial exposure attempts is a good idea, you shouldn't use relaxation with exposure and response prevention for OCD. That's because one of the crucial lessons is that your anxiety will come down if and only if you give exposure enough time. Furthermore, some of those with OCD actually start to use relaxation as a compulsive ritual itself. Thus it's fine if you want to practise a little relaxation for anxieties not related to your OCD, but don't use it with exposure and response prevention.

Preparing for exposure and response prevention

Prior to actual exposure and response prevention, you may find it useful to alter your compulsive rituals in ways that start to disrupt and alter their influence over you. Methods for initiating this assault on compulsions include:

- **Delay performing your ritual when you first feel the urge.** For example, if you have a strong compulsion to wipe the doorknobs and the phones with an anti-bacterial cleaner, try putting it off for at least 30 minutes. The next day, try to delay acting on your urge for 45 minutes.

- **Carry out your compulsion at a much slower pace than usual.** For example, if you feel compelled to arrange items in a perfect row, go ahead and do it, but lay them out with excruciating slowness.

- **Change your compulsion in some way.** If it's a ritual, change the number of times that you do it. If it involves a sequence of checking all the door locks in the house, try doing them in a completely different order to your usual order.

Carrying out exposure and response prevention for OCD

Ingrid worries constantly about getting ill from dirt, germs, and pesticides. Whenever she thinks that she may have come into contact with any of these to the slightest degree, she feels compelled to wash her hands thoroughly, first with an abrasive soap to remove the dirty layer of skin, and then with anti-bacterial soap to kill the germs. Unfortunately, this means her hands become cracked, sore, and bleeding. When she goes out into public she wears gloves to hide the self-inflicted damage. Not only that, she's discovering that her hand washing consumes increasing amounts of time. Her 15-minute breaks at work are too short to complete her hand-washing. Ingrid finally decides to do something about her problem when her supervisor at work tells her that she must take shorter breaks. Ingrid prepares for her exposure and response prevention exercise by doing the following for a week:

- She delays washing her hands for 30 minutes when she feels the urge. Later she delays washing for 45 minutes.

- She changes to using an ordinary soap.

Ingrid is surprised to find that these changes make her hand-washing urges a little less frequent, but they haven't exactly disappeared, and they continue to cause considerable distress. She needs to muster the courage to do full exposure and response prevention.

First, she approaches Helen, a trusted friend, for help. She tells Helen about her problem and asks her to support and encourage her through the exercises. Then she makes a tower of fear for her exposure and response prevention that includes touching the following 'dirty dozen':

- Toilet seats (with her bare hands). Anxiety: 99
- Cans of pesticide. Anxiety: 92
- Her cat's litter tray. Anxiety: 90
- Motor oil. Anxiety: 87
- Dirty carpets. Anxiety: 86
- Doorknobs. Anxiety: 80
- Handrails on an escalator. Anxiety: 78
- The wheel of a car driven by someone else. Anxiety: 72
- Unwashed fruits and vegetables. Anxiety: 70
- The seat of a chair that a sick person sat on. Anxiety: 67
- The seat of a chair that a healthy person sat on. Anxiety: 60
- A telephone receiver that someone else has used. Anxiety: 53

Helen helps Ingrid with her tower of fear by having her start with the easiest building block – touching a telephone receiver that someone else used. She encourages Ingrid to do this a number of times and to resist the urge to wash her hands. After an hour and a half, the urge to wash drops significantly. The next day, Helen encourages Ingrid to tackle the next building block.

Each day, if Ingrid has succeeded on the previous day, Helen helps Ingrid move on to the next new building block. When she gets to touching the cat's litter tray, Ingrid balks at first. Helen says that she won't make Ingrid do it, but she thinks it just may help her. In other words, she urges her on. The cat litter tray takes many attempts. Finally, Ingrid manages to touch it and stay with it. However, it takes a total of three hours of repeatedly attempting and finally touching the litter tray numerous times for as long as ten minutes each time for her anxiety to come down by half.

At times, exposure and response prevention can take a while, so make sure that you have plenty of time set aside. In Ingrid's case, the final two items didn't require as much effort, because her earlier work had enabled her to reduce the power that her compulsions had over her.

If you can't do this on your own or with a friend, please consult a professional for help.

To make it less likely that you get stuck on exposure and response prevention, you may want to consult Chapter 5 and work through it carefully. Pay particular attention to the section on rethinking risk. Usually, those with OCD overestimate the odds of catastrophic outcomes if they halt their compulsions, and this chapter can help you recalculate the odds.

Chasing Rainbows

Sometimes, people come to us asking for a quick fix for their anxiety problems. It's as though they think that we have some magic wand that we wave over them and everything will get better. That would be so nice, but it isn't realistic.

Other people hope that, with help, they'll rid themselves of all anxiety – another misconception. Some anxiety helps prepare you for action, warn you of danger, and mobilise your resources. The only people who are completely without anxiety are unconscious or dead.

Overcoming anxiety requires effort and some discomfort. There's no way around that. No magic wand. But we know that those who undertake the challenge, make the effort, and suffer the discomfort are rewarded with new confidence and a vastly improved quality of life.

Chapter 9

Simply Simplifying Your Life

. . . .

In This Chapter

▶ Discovering what's really important to you

▶ Prioritising goals

▶ Getting help from others

▶ Saying no

. . . .

*P*hil answers the phone again for the third time since sitting down for dinner with his family. 'Oh, sure', he agrees, 'I can help referee the boys' football match this Saturday.' His wife groans, 'I thought you were going to help my brother move this weekend, and our house is a mess. Remember? We were going to clean it up together.'

'Don't forget, Dad, you promised me you'd come and sell raffle tickets door to door,' whines his daughter, 'and I need a lift to the shopping centre in 15 minutes.' Phil's stomach starts to burn. He grabs an antacid from his pocket and sucks on it. 'We can drop you off on the way to the supermarket and pick you up when we're finished', Phil responds, feeling harassed.

Phil and his wife both work full time at demanding jobs. Their two kids are heavily into many activities. Phil tries to be a good dad, but sometimes he just gets tired. Does this sound like your family? Do you have too much to do? If so, your stress and anxiety probably increase when demands take over your life. In this chapter, we describe four sound strategies for simplifying your life:

✔ **Exploring the things you value:** Take our quiz to clarify the things you value and decide what areas in life are meaningful to you, and then find out how to devote more time and energy to those and less to other things.

✔ **Prioritising and setting goals:** After you figure out what's most important, give these goals top priority to help you get what you want.

✔ **Discovering the importance of delegating:** Doing all the work yourself can be cumbersome and even impossible, so letting somebody else do it can improve the quality of your life – and theirs.

✔ **Discovering the power of NO:** It's only a two-letter word, but saying no when you need to can make your life much more manageable.

Evaluating What's Important Versus What's Not

Everyone would like to have it all, and some book titles promise that you can. It's a seductive idea. Who wouldn't want everything possible from life?

- An abundance of friends
- Adventure
- Career success
- A close family
- Good health
- Happiness
- Leisure time
- Power
- Recognition
- Rewarding hobbies
- Security
- Spirituality
- Successful, happy children
- True, lasting love
- Wealth

Nice list. No doubt a few exceptionally lucky people do almost have it all. But this book deals with the real world, and the real world throws the unexpected at you. Life also provides only a limited amount of time within which to manage all that we need to do. Thus most people must make tough choices on how to use their time.

Prioritising choices: Not having it all

We can help you prioritise your choices. Take our quiz to clarify the things you value and then compare the results with how you actually spend your time. You may be surprised to see there's a mismatch between what you value and what you spend your time doing.

Look over the list of things that you may value, which follows. Circle the eight that matter the most to you. Then go back and underline the top three.

Achievement	Leisure time
Art	Looking good
Cleaning up the environment	Loving partner
Close friends	Mental or physical stimulation
Competition	Money
Creativity	Pleasure
Donating time/money	Political activism
Economic security	Predictability
Entertainment	Recognition
Expensive possessions	Recreation
Family life	Risk taking
Good food	Safety/security
Having happy kids	Satisfying work
Health	Showing kindness
Honesty	Spirituality
Independence	Successful career
Influencing others	Variety
Intellectual pursuits	Zany activities

Doing what's important to you

Which of the things that you value stand out as most important for you? Now review a month in your life. You can do this by keeping an activity time log as follows:

1. **Write down every activity and how long you spend on it.**

   Don't worry about trivial details like washing your hands (unless it's part of an obsessive-compulsive problem).

2. **If you forget to write down your activities for a few hours, try to fill your log in from memory.**

   You can even record your activities once a day before bedtime. Perfect accuracy is not important.

3. When the month is over, total up the total hours spent on each type of activity.

What really matters is how much time you devote to what you value. How do the activities that you value match up with the amount of time that you spend on them?

Grace, for example, feels stressed and anxious and that she never has enough time for anything. Grace completes the quiz to clarify the things she values and chooses close friends, satisfying work, and family life as her most highly prized activities. Then Grace tracks her activities in a time log for a month. The following list shows how Grace spends her time that month:

- ✔ Work: 205 hours
- ✔ Watching television: 60 hours
- ✔ Eating meals: 45 hours
- ✔ Commuting to work and child daycare: 44 hours
- ✔ Showering and getting ready in the morning: 30 hours
- ✔ Meal preparation: 30 hours
- ✔ Taking kids to sports and lessons: 24 hours
- ✔ Housework: 22 hours
- ✔ Shopping/errands: 10 hours
- ✔ Exercise: 4 hours
- ✔ Household accounts: 3 hours
- ✔ Time with friends: 2 hours
- ✔ Time alone with husband: 1 hour

As she reviews her time log, Grace realises she works a 50-hour week in her job as a financial planner. Although the job provides challenge, satisfaction, and a good income, Grace doesn't find it particularly meaningful. She's appalled to realise that she spends a mere 30 minutes per week with her friends. Even worse, she spends almost no time alone with her husband. Her time with her children consists of shuttling them to and from child-minder and various activities. Hardly what she considers quality family time.

Shame and dismay flood Grace as she notices that television consumes more of her time than any single activity outside of work. She knows that she's not living the life that she imagined she would. So Grace decides to do something different.

Ranking Priorities

Try not to let yourself feel ashamed and dismayed, like Grace did, when you review what you are doing, comparing your activities with the things you value, and perhaps find that your life has strayed off course. The fact is, most people discover that the way they spend their time differs considerably from the things they profess to value. Nevertheless, if you want to, you can turn things around.

If you completed a time log, compare what you actually do against the things you value. If a discrepancy exists, prioritise and set goals. Simplify your life. Make sure that your goals are specific and obtainable. Don't make goals like 'I'll be happier' or 'I'll save more money' because these are too vague. Instead, state specific ideas for increasing your happiness, such as going swimming once a week or playing tennis twice a month, or reading at least one book for pleasure per month. You can arrange to have £100 per month automatically withdrawn from your account to go into savings and agree with friends that that you will go out for an evening on the first Monday of each month.

Grace starts by poring over her time log for the past month. Television viewing jumps out as the first candidate for the chopping block. She decides to limit her television viewing and to improve the quality of her family time. She sets the following concrete goals:

- ✔ I will only watch my favourite news shows that come on after the kids are put to bed.

- ✔ Friday night will be family night. We'll get a takeaway, play games, and talk.

- ✔ Once a month, we'll get a babysitter, and my husband and I will go out for the evening.

- ✔ Two Saturdays per month, we'll choose a family activity such as bowling or going out somewhere.

Grace feels good about her new goals and priorities. However, she realises that she still works too many hours and has not found a way to include friends in her life. Since the kids were born, she's lost contact with most of her good friends. Looking at her schedule, she wonders what to do.

Delegating Tasks to Free Up Extra Time

Many people with anxiety feel they must take all the responsibility for their jobs, the care of their families, and their homes. Unless they have a role in everything, they worry things may not get done. And if someone else takes over a task, they fear the result will fall short of their standards.

Grace works many long hours and still feels the need to cook, clean, transport her kids, and do most of the household errands. Sometimes her husband offers to do the washing or cooking, but she turns him down, thinking that he'll only mess it up. But when Grace makes the decision to reorganise her life, she knows that she'll have to start delegating. She ponders what, how, who, and when. Talking to some close friends, she discovers they are as stuck and dissatisfied as her. Remembering some brainstorming techniques learned at a business seminar, she invites a couple of her friends over with their partners and suggests they all work together on the ideas. They come up with tasks that can be delegated, to share out the onerous workload. See the following list to find out what they came up with:

- ✔ **Take the risk of letting husband do some laundry and cooking.** If he makes a mess of it, Grace can show him how to improve next time.

- ✔ **Employ a cleaner to do the ironing and the more time-consuming domestic chores.** While it may cost a bit, Grace's long working hours earn her more than enough money to cover it.

- ✔ **Buy good quality pre-prepared foods, with minimal or preferably no additives, that just need to be placed in the oven to cook.**

- ✔ **The whole family can spend one hour a week in a concentrated, joint cleaning effort.** Her husband suggests that if everyone does the cleaning at the same time, with specific delegated tasks, it may even be fun.

- ✔ **Grace's secretary will take on some more responsibilities, including dealing with some client phone calls and scheduling Grace's appointments.** Grace realises that because she so seldom delegates, her secretary has quite a bit of free time. Grace also discovers that her secretary is much happier with the additional responsibility and challenges.

- ✔ **Employ someone to come in monthly and do the heavy, time-consuming work in the garden.** Grace's husband says that he doesn't mind doing some of the work, but employing someone would give them more time together.

- ✔ **Read *Organizing For Dummies* by Eileen Roth and Elizabeth Miles (Wiley).** It's got some great tips on how to save time and effort and get organised. If you don't want to go down the route of hiring outside help, this book can help you do it yourself in less time. When you're organised, tasks go more smoothly and faster.

We realise a number of these ideas cost money. Not always as much as you may think, but still they do cost something. Partly it's a matter of how highly you rate money on your priority list. Balance money against time for the things that you value.

However, not all families can consider such options. While not all these options have financial implications, why not get creative? Ask your friends, colleagues, and family for ideas on how to delegate. It may change your life.

Come up with two tasks that you can delegate to someone else. They don't need to cost money, just relieve one or more of your burdens in a way that can save you time and give you more energy to spend on what you enjoy.

Just Saying No

We have one more idea. Say no. If you're anxious, you may have trouble standing up for your rights. Anxiety often prevents people from expressing their feelings and needs. When that happens, resentment joins anxiety and leads to frustration and anger. Furthermore, if you can't say no, other people can purposefully or inadvertently take advantage of you. You no longer own your time and your life.

Grace agrees to do nearly all that anyone asks of her. When her boss asks her to work late at the last minute, she always agrees. Even if working late impinges on important plans, she rarely expresses unwillingness. She also finds it difficult to hang up on annoying cold-call telephone sales people. She gives a few pounds to every charity request, even if she's never heard of the organisation. She drives other people's children more than any of the other parents who are in the lift-sharing scheme. When her children need last-minute help on homework projects because of their own procrastination, she pitches in despite her own fatigue and better judgement.

If you're a little like Grace, we have some suggestions for learning how to say no. Realise it will take you some time to incorporate this new habit. You've probably been agreeing to fulfil everyone's requests for many years, so it will take a while to do something different.

First, notice the situations in which you find yourself agreeing when you don't really want to. Does it happen mostly at work, with family, with friends, or with strangers? When people ask you to do something, try the following:

- ✔ **Validate the person's request or desire.** For example, if someone asks you if you would mind dropping off something at the post office on your way home from work, say, 'I know it's more convenient for you if I drop it off . . .' This will give you more time to consider whether you really want to do it.

- ✔ **After you make up your mind, look the person who's making the request in the eye.** You don't need to rush your response.

- ✔ **Give a brief explanation, especially if it's a friend or family member.** However, remember that you really don't owe anyone an explanation; it's only good manners. You can say that you'd like to help out, but it just isn't possible, or you can even simply state that you really would rather not.

> ✔ **Be explicit that you if are choosing to do what you've been asked, this does not mean you are setting a precedent that you will always follow.** You can always add 'I can't do this regularly, though.'
>
> ✔ **Be clear that you cannot or will not do what you've been asked.** It's a fundamental human right to say no.
>
> ✔ **If you do fall into the old habit of saying yes, contact the person the next day and explain that having thought about it, you realise it just isn't feasible.** Allow yourself a second bite at the cherry, rather than telling yourself that now you have agreed, you are saddled with that decision.

Grace answers the phone and a double-glazing salesperson cheerfully begins his spiel. He talks so quickly that Grace can't speak without interrupting him. Then she realises that she has the right to interrupt. After all, he's interrupting her dinner. So she musters up her courage and declares, 'Thank you for calling. I'm just not interested.' The salesperson goes right on and says, 'Can I ask you why not?' She responds 'No!' and hangs up the phone. Her husband and children look on in amazement.

When you say no to bosses, colleagues, friends, or family members, they may be temporarily unhappy with you. If you find yourself overreacting to their displeasure, it may be due to an anxiety-provoking assumption. See Chapter 6 for more information on these.

Chapter 10

Getting Physical

*A*t 50 years of age, **Hope** continues to struggle with tension and feels on edge much of the time. Of course, she's doing much better than she was a few years ago, before she went to a therapist for her panic attacks. At that time, she'd been taking quite a few days off work due to her anxiety disorder, and she averaged four panic attacks per week. Her therapist taught her many of the strategies that we discuss in Chapters 5, 6, 7, 8, and 16. These techniques have virtually eliminated her panic attacks, but Hope still seems to feel worked up most of the time.

Hope tries several different medications but doesn't like the side effects. She also notices that she's gaining weight, which is common among women of her age group. A friend persuades her to join a gym. Along with the membership come four sessions with a personal trainer. Within a matter of six weeks, Hope discovers a passion for exercise. Her mood improves; her anxiety and stress decrease. She even begins to lose a few pounds, and she feels great. Others notice and comment; this increases her motivation and efforts.

In this chapter, we review the many benefits of exercise. A solid exercise regime not only helps you overcome your anxiety, but it also improves your health, appearance, and sense of wellbeing. The catch for most people lies in finding the motivation and time to make exercise a part of their routine. We help you find the motivation and show you how to develop a workable plan. We also guide you through the various exercise programme options. The best option for you primarily depends upon your personal goals and state of health.

Ready Steady . . . Exorcise!

Please excuse our pun: We're not advising that you attempt to exorcise demons or perform hocus pocus, but like a good spring cleaning, exercise can banish the cobwebs and cast out the cloudy thinking and inertia that may accompany anxiety.

Exercise reduces anxiety. The harder and longer you work at it, whether you're playing sport, swimming, jogging, walking, gardening, or even climbing the stairs, the less anxious you'll be. Exercise instils a new-found sense of confidence while blowing away anxiety's cloud. With sufficient exercise, you'll notice your attitude change from negative to positive.

Exercise reduces anxiety in several ways:

✔ Exercise helps to rid your body of the excess adrenaline that increases anxiety and arousal.

✔ Working out increases your body's production of *endorphins* – substances that reduce pain and create a mild, natural sense of wellbeing.

✔ Exercise also helps to release muscle tension and frustrations.

Of course, everyone has felt they should exercise more. Most people realise that exercise has some sorts of benefits for their health, but not everyone knows how extensive these benefits can be.

✔ Researchers have found that exercise decreases

- Anxiety
- Bad cholesterol
- Blood pressure
- Chronic pain
- Depression
- Low back pain

✔ Researchers have also found that exercise decreases the risk of

- Breast cancer
- Colon cancer
- Diabetes
- Falling, especially among the elderly
- Heart attacks
- Strokes

✔ Research also supports the claim that exercise increases

- A sense of balance

- Endurance

- Energy

- Flexibility

- The functioning of the immune system

- Good cholesterol

- Lung capacity

- Mental sharpness

- A sense of wellbeing

Wow! With such extensive, positive effects on anxiety, health, and wellbeing, why isn't everyone exercising? Millions of people do. Unfortunately, millions do not. The reason is both simple and complex. For the most part, people hit a brick wall when it comes to finding the motivation to exercise and especially for sustaining it. They complain about not having the time and being too embarrassed, too old, too fat, and too tired to exercise. But if our list of benefits appeals to you, the next section, 'Don't Wait for Willpower – Just Do It', may help you muster the motivation.

Before beginning an exercise programme, you should first check with your GP. This is especially true if you're over 40, overweight, or have any known health problems. Your GP can tell you about any cautions, limitations, or restrictions that you should consider. Also, if during brief exercise you experience chest pain, extreme shortness of breath, nausea, or dizziness, stop at once and consult your GP immediately.

Don't Wait for Willpower – Just Do It

Have you ever thought that you just don't have the willpower to undertake an exercise programme? You may be surprised to discover that we don't believe in willpower. That's right. *Willpower* is merely a word, an idea; it's not real.

Your brain doesn't have a special structure that contains so-called willpower. It's not something that you have a set quantity of and that you can't do anything about. The reason why people believe that they don't have willpower is that they merely don't do what they think they should. But reasons other than willpower exist to account for the lack of effort.

People fail to undertake projects for several kinds of reasons:

- ✔ **Distorted thinking:** Your mind may tell you things like 'I just don't have the time', 'I'm too tired', 'It isn't worth the effort', or 'I'll look stupid compared to others who are in better shape than me'.

- ✔ **Lack of reward:** This problem comes about when you fail to set up a plan for rewarding new efforts. You may believe that exercise will cost you something in terms of leisure time, rest, or more profitable work. In some ways, this is true. That's why you need to set up a plan for reinforcing your efforts.

- ✔ **Environmental obstacles:** Perhaps you don't know of a good place for exercising, or the weather in your area isn't conducive. Maybe you have young children that you need to take care of. You'll need to find ways around these obstacles.

- ✔ **Insufficient support:** We all need support sometimes. Exercising alone can be tough for anyone, especially if your partner doesn't want to participate.

Defeating defeatism

If you're waiting for motivation to come knocking at your door, you may be in for a long wait. Not many people wake up with a burst of new enthusiasm for starting an exercise programme. Like the commercial says, 'Just do it.' That's because motivation frequently follows action; if you think otherwise, you're putting the cart before the horse. Thinking that you should wait for the motivation before taking action is one of the top ten defeatist ideas.

We list the top ten most defeatist ideas with arguments against them in Table 10-1. Look these over carefully to see which, if any, may be hindering your decision to exercise. Ponder both sides carefully.

Table 10-1	The Top Ten Defeatist Ideas
Defeatist Ideas	*Debunking Defeatist Ideas*
I don't have the motivation. When inspiration comes to me, I'll start exercising.	Motivation follows action, not the other way round. Regular exercise feels great eventually, but that often takes time.
I don't have time.	Time is only a matter of priorities. Exercising for 30 minutes, three times a week, will be a good start.

Defeatist Ideas	*Debunking Defeatist Ideas*
I'm too tired.	I'm tired much of the time because I don't exercise! Exercise increases energy and stamina.
I'm too old for exercise.	No-one is ever too old to exercise. GPs say that it's good at every age; even people over the age of 80 can benefit from exercise. They just have to start slowly and set realistic goals.
I'll look silly compared with the people who are in better condition.	Everyone starts from somewhere. If I'm too embarrassed, I can start at home. I can join others when I start to get somewhere.
It's too expensive to go to the gym.	Compared with the costs of poor health, it's cheap. Anyway, I can exercise without going to a gym.
It's not worth the effort.	It may feel that way sometimes, but the benefits are indisputable.
I have too much to do at work. I can't take time away for something silly like exercise.	Studies show that people who exercise regularly miss fewer days at work. Plus they're probably more productive as well.
I don't like exercise.	So far, I haven't enjoyed it, but I don't have to enjoy everything that's good for me. I don't like my annual check up, but I go through with it, and I can always try different kinds of exercise; maybe I will find one that I do like.
I'm just not an exerciser. It's not who I am.	With all the benefits that exercise holds for me, I need to work out. I don't have to think of myself as some sportsperson, I just need to exercise three or four times a week.

If you have one or more of these defeatist ideas running around in your head, perhaps you agree with our counter-arguments. If you don't agree with our counter-arguments, see whether you can develop your own way of countering defeatist thoughts and ideas. Chapter 3 has many ideas for overcoming the thoughts that cause resistance to change. If you find motivation elusive, you're not exactly the first person in the world to have that problem.

Willpower is a misnomer; you simply need to tackle the thoughts that stand in your way and then try our other ways to develop motivation, which are explained in the rest of this chapter.

Rewarding yourself for exercise

Psychologists have known for decades that people usually do more of what they find rewarding and less of what they find unpleasant whenever they can. That fact may sound like stating the obvious to you. Nevertheless, ignoring the importance of rewards is easy when trying to get started on an exercise programme.

If you're out of shape right now, exercise may feel more unpleasant than pleasant, at least at the beginning. During or after your workout, you may be out of breath, your muscles may ache, and you may have soreness for a few days or even longer. Reminding yourself of the benefits of exercise can help, but let's face it: The benefits don't accrue until you've been working out a while.

A large number of the problems that people struggle with involve difficulty in balancing short-term payoffs versus long-term benefits and costs. Don't you think so? Consider the common bad habits presented in Table 10-2. The greater tendency towards immediate gratification overshadows any consideration of the detrimental effects that arise over the long haul.

Table 10-2	The Effects of Bad Habits	
Example	*Short-term Payoff*	*Long-term Result*
Alcohol abuse	Drinking usually feels better than abstinence.	Alcohol can kill you.
Smoking	Smokers claim that smoking relaxes them.	A wide range of health problems.
Overeating	People wrestling with weight find eating satisfying.	Many health problems.
Drug abuse	Many so-called recreational drugs feel good.	Permanent body and brain damage.
Spending problems	Spending money is usually fun.	Savings and retirement suffer badly.

Exercise involves the same problem with balancing short- versus long-term payoffs, but the payoffs are only apparent after consistent, long-term participation. At first, exercise more often than not feels lousy, whereas, eventually, for those who keep up the routine, a daily workout improves your health and sense of wellbeing. Unfortunately, people have a hard time doing what may feel unpleasant in the short run, even if benefits await them over time.

However, you can work your way around this dilemma: Set up your own personal reward system for exercising. For example, give yourself ten points for each time that you exercise for 30 minutes or more. After you accumulate 100 points, indulge yourself with a treat such as a new outfit, going out for dinner at a nice restaurant, planning a special weekend, or setting aside a whole day to spend on your favourite hobby. Over time, as exercise becomes a little more pleasant (which it will!), up the ante to 200 points before you treat yourself.

Eventually, you'll find that exercise becomes rewarding in its own right, and you won't need to reward yourself as a means of instilling the necessary motivation. As the pain of an out-of-shape body lessens and endurance increases, you'll discover other rewards from exercise as well, such as:

- ✔ It can be a great time to think about solutions to problems.
- ✔ You can plan out the day or week while you exercise.
- ✔ Some people report increased creative thoughts during exercise.
- ✔ You may get a great feeling from the sense of accomplishment.

The desperado's self-starter plan

If you really want to exercise but still haven't started, try what we call the *desperado's self-starter plan* to test whether you really want to start exercising. The desperado's self-starter plan has just a few simple steps:

- ✔ Write out five cheques for an amount of money that it would hurt to lose, but not so much that it would blow your whole budget – perhaps £10 or £20 each.

- ✔ Look up the address of some organisation that you don't like, perhaps a political party or a local organisation that you love to hate.

- ✔ Write a letter in support of this organisation and sign it.

- ✔ Hand the stamped letters with the cheques to a highly trusted friend. Tell your friend that you will report each week for five weeks whether you exercised three or more times that week. If you did not, ask that your letter be posted.

Ouch! Are we serious? Yes. We have tried this strategy with a variety of clients in the past. Trust us: It's a rare person who allows those letters to actually end up in the post.

The desperado's self-starter plan usually works best for relatively short-term motivational requirements that last six weeks or less. Don't rely on it for long-term solutions. The good news is that exercise programmes often become self-sustaining within four or five weeks of consistent effort.

Because exercise often doesn't feel good at the beginning, setting up a self-reward system sometimes helps a great deal; later, other rewards are likely to kick in.

However, if you find that even a self-reward programme doesn't quite do the trick, what else can you do? We have one more idea that's a bit more ferocious – the desperado's self-starter plan. (See 'The desperado's self-starter plan' sidebar in this chapter.)

Jumping over the barriers to exercise

Sometimes people struggle with starting to exercise because of a few personal or environmental obstacles. You want to exercise, but inconveniences just get in the way, such as:

- Weather that's too cold and or unsettled for jogging
- Overly crowded municipal gyms in your area, where equipment is always in use
- Prohibitively expensive private gym membership
- Dangerous localities that feel unsafe for walking or jogging
- A lack of exercise equipment and no money to buy it

Perhaps surprisingly, the real problem with these obstacles lies in your mindset and not in the hindrances themselves. These are merely inconveniences, hassles, little problems waiting to be solved, rather than concrete blockades.

Consider turning an unused room or space in your home into a workout space. Make the room as exercise-friendly as possible. You may want to have a music system or headphones, a television to watch, or simply a book to read while you are pedalling away on your exercise bike. In addition, you can stock your room with simple, relatively inexpensive equipment; you don't have to spend a fortune on exercise equipment. Consider using:

- Skipping ropes
- Cans of soup or plastic bottles of water instead of hand weights
- A stair or some bricks for stepping exercises
- An inexpensive yoga mat
- Reasonably priced exercise equipment

Think creatively. Car boot or garage sales are a good bet for finding reasonably priced exercise equipment. Sometimes it takes a little thought to find the right place, time, and type of equipment that you want to use. But realise that you can solve the problem, and your solution doesn't have to be a perfect one. Something is most definitely better than nothing, and every little really does help.

Encouraging encouragement

Although social supports aren't absolutely essential, many people find that company can increase motivation to exercise. Other people can give you encouragement and provide someone interesting to talk to. You can obtain social support in various ways:

- ✔ **Two's company:** If you know someone who has talked about wanting to exercise, you have an instant support system. If you don't, try discussing your problem with your friends. If they don't want to exercise, perhaps they know someone else who does. Leave no stone unturned.

- ✔ **Taking a class:** All kinds of exercise classes are available at the local adult education colleges, local council facilities and sports centres.

- ✔ **Joining a gym:** You'll find like-minded people at health clubs or gyms. Classes often take place as well as individual work-out facilities. Many of the members are new to exercise or have a hard time sticking to it after they start up a programme, just like you. That's especially true in January!

- ✔ **Getting a personal trainer:** It sounds expensive, doesn't it? Personal trainers do cost, but they can help you design a programme and push you to stick with it. You may be able to reduce the cost by getting a personal trainer for yourself and a friend for less than the two of you would pay separately. You'll find that after four or five weeks, you won't need your trainer often, or perhaps even at all.

The bottom line is that humans are social animals. Undertaking a new but difficult enterprise is easier if you have support system, which is probably available to you if you give it some thought.

Fitting in Your Fitness Programme

Today, people work increasingly longer hours, so it's tempting to think that not enough hours exist in the day for exercise. Of course, we covered the distorted belief that 'I don't have time to exercise' in Table 10-1 earlier in this chapter. However, even though you may have come to the realisation that you have the time and that it's all a matter of priorities, you won't find the time unless you actually plan it in.

That's right: You have to scrutinise your schedule seriously and work exercise into your life. Perhaps your job offers flexitime, whereby you can choose to come in an hour later and stay later two or three times a week to have time to exercise in the morning, or perhaps you can exercise twice at the weekend and find just one time after work during the week.

Conventional advice suggests that you should do some kind of vigorous exercise for half an hour or more at least three times a week. Perhaps you can fit exercise in at the weekend and find a third time during the week by getting creative. It isn't all that difficult. For example:

- **Parking at a distance:** Park your car about a 20-minute brisk walk away from your place of work once or twice a week. Choose the spaces in the supermarket car park that are furthest from the entrance.

- **Taking the stairs:** If you often take the lift up five or six floors to work, try a brisk walk up the stairs several times a day instead.

- **Exercising during your breaks:** If you get a couple of 10- or 15-minute breaks at work, try going for a brisk walk rather than standing around the coffee machine. Two or three 10-minute periods of exercise do you the same amount of good that one 20- or 30-minute period does.

- **Walk rather than drive:** Consider each time you get into your car whether it would be feasible to walk.

- **Get a dog!** Many people are spurred into exercise by the feeling they have to take the dog for a daily walk. They report that they then become part of a friendly community of dog-walkers, which makes the exercise an enjoyable social outing for both owner and dog.

Selecting an Exercise – Whatever Turns You On

Choosing the type of exercise that works best for you depends in part on what goals you have. Almost any exercise can reduce anxiety somewhat. However, you're bound to find that you like certain types of exercise more than others. Because any exercise has benefits, we recommend that you start with exercise that seems most appealing to you. Although the array of exercise possibilities is almost infinite, some of the most popular forms of exercise are aerobics, weight training, and yoga.

Pumping up your heart and lungs

One of the best ways to alleviate anxiety is to engage in *aerobic* exercise (also known as *cardiovascular* exercise). *Aerobic* means 'with oxygen', and it refers to the kind of energetic, vigorous exercise that increases your intake of oxygen and thus shapes up your heart and lungs. Aerobic exercise also lowers blood pressure, reduces bad cholesterol while raising your good cholesterol, and builds up your energy and endurance.

Aerobic exercise involves working your large muscles in rhythmic, repetitive actions and lasts for more than a few minutes. To get the most benefit, you should keep at it for 20 or 30 minutes, although two or three 10-minute periods work pretty well too. Types of aerobic exercise include

- Badminton
- Basketball
- Cycling
- Jogging
- Rowing
- Skating
- Squash
- Swimming
- Tennis
- Volleyball
- Walking briskly

With aerobic exercise, you want to feel winded but still be able to say a five- or six-word sentence without gasping for another breath – an indication that your heart and lungs are working hard enough to improve their condition, but not so hard that you pass out.

To be precise, you can get an inexpensive heart monitor and track your pulse, or to get a general idea, you can take your pulse yourself by putting your index finger on the artery in your neck that's just below your chin and next to your Adam's apple. The artery isn't hard to find because you'll feel the rhythmic pumping of blood through it with your fingers. Your *pulse* tells you how fast or slow your heart is beating. Look at a clock with a second hand and, with your finger on your artery, count the beats that occur within 15 seconds and multiply that number by four to find out the number of beats per minute, otherwise known as your pulse rate.

A basic formula is available to figure out your ideal heart rate when exercising. Essentially, you subtract your age from 220 and multiply the result by a percentage that depends upon your fitness level.

If you're a healthy beginner, but in poor shape, subtract your age from 220 and multiply the result by 0.5. For example, if you're 35 years old and haven't exercised since your school days, you calculate your initial target heart rate when exercising as follows:

$$220 - 35 = 185 \times 0.5 = 92.5$$

If on the other hand, you're in moderately good shape, multiply the result by 0.6. For example, if you're 65 years old, have been fairly active, and have your GP's approval for exercise, you would calculate your target zone this way:

$$220 - 65 = 155 \times 0.6 = 93.0$$

Finally, if you're already in very good condition, you can multiply the result by 0.8. For example, if you're 53 years old and have been exercising vigorously for quite some time, you would calculate your target zone this way:

$$220 - 53 = 167 \times 0.8 = 133.6$$

When you're exercising vigorously, your heart rate is likely to go over your target rate. When that happens, it's time to slow down and bring your pulse back into the training zone.

Everyone should have regular physical check-ups. If you're over 40 or have any kind of health concerns, be sure to consult your GP for help in determining your fitness level and target heart rate. At the other end of the scale, if you exercise for hours each day to the point of total exhaustion, this is unlikely to be good for you, and we suggest you discuss this with your GP.

Lifting your way out of anxiety

Weight training mainly builds strength, and it may not reduce anxiety as well as aerobic exercise, but some people believe that it helps. They say that their confidence improves and tension reduces.

Probably the easiest way to do weight training is by using dumb-bells, barbells, or weight machines. However, you can obtain reasonable strength gains from some inexpensive resistance machines as well as rubber exercise bands, and even exercises that do not need equipment, such as:

- ✔ Crunches
- ✔ Lunges
- ✔ Press-ups
- ✔ Squats

You should know that strength and weight training require some knowledge. Before you train with weights, we recommend that you consult a trainer or purchase a book, such as *Weight Training For Dummies,* 3rd Edition, by Liz Neporent, Suzanne Schlosberg, and Shirley J. Archer (Wiley). Then you can start pumping and lifting your anxiety up and away.

Yearning to try yoga?

You'd almost have to live in a monastery not to have heard of yoga nowadays. No-one knows for sure when yoga actually began, but it's been around for at least 3,000 to 5,000 years. The many types and versions of yoga involve a series of poses that you hold for perhaps 30 seconds to a couple of minutes. Various stories abound about the origins of yoga, but most people believe that it developed in India and was practised by Buddhist monks.

For many, yoga has a spiritual component. Others practise it merely as an exercise. You can do either or both; there's no fixed rule about how to practise yoga.

Yoga has some interesting benefits. First, it can be quite relaxing and anxiety alleviating. It also blends nicely with a practice known as *mindfulness,* described in Chapter 16. As a combination, yoga and mindfulness can become a powerful tool against anxiety. Secondly, yoga has positive physiological effects, such as increased strength, flexibility, and balance. Certain versions of yoga can even be somewhat aerobic.

However, perhaps you think of yoga as tying your body up like a human pretzel, or maybe you've seen pictures of people sitting on the floor with their eyes closed and thought that yoga looks more like sleep than exercise. Both of these ideas are myths, as we can personally attest.

A couple of years ago, Laura (one of the authors of this book) started dabbling in yoga. She came home and extolled the virtues of yoga to Charles (another author of this book). He writes 'I supported her new interest, but I knew it wasn't for me. After all, I'm 6 feet, 3 inches tall, and at that time I had as much flexibility in my body as a bronze statue. I imagined looking like a total buffoon or worse.

How about exercise and panic?

Some people fear that exercise may set off panic attacks. In part, that's because exercise does produce a variety of bodily symptoms, such as increased heart rate, and those with panic attacks sometimes respond to such symptoms with alarm. However, if you undertake exercise gradually, it can serve as a graded exposure task, as discussed in Chapter 8. In other words, it can be an effective treatment approach for panic.

In addition, exercise can cause a build up of lactic acid, which does seem to trigger panic attacks in a few people, although the actual risk is somewhat controversial. However, over the long run, exercise also improves your body's ability to rid itself of lactic acid. Therefore, again, we recommend that if you fear you'll have panic attacks as a result of exercise, simply take it slowly. If you find exercise absolutely intolerable, stop exercising for a while or use other strategies in this book for reducing your panic attack frequency before going back to exercise.

After a few months, Laura urged me to join her. I said that may happen . . . when pigs fly. She persisted. (She persists when she's really right about something.) Eventually, when at a professional conference together, she suggested that we arrange a private lesson with the spa connected to the hotel that we were staying in. I decided that perhaps a private lesson wouldn't be quite so humiliating, and I could show her once and for all that I wasn't going to like yoga, much less be capable of doing it.

Well, I was wrong. Although my body didn't bend like a pretzel, the instructor showed me how to honour any restrictive signals that my body gave me, and he pointed out that yoga is non-competitive – you don't have to look great. Today, both of us enjoy yoga and find it quite relaxing. We've experienced increased flexibility, balance, strength, and calm.'

Like weight training, yoga requires a little knowledge. You can sign up for a beginner's class, read a book like *Yoga For Dummies* by Georg Feuerstein and Larry Payne (Wiley), or check out one of a variety of videos, such as *Basic Yoga Workout For Dummies* with Susan Ivanhoe (Wiley). We think that your investigation will be worth the effort. Yoga just may surprise you.

Chapter 11

Sleep, Sweet Sleep

• •

• •

Does this little script from the wee small-hours sound familiar? It's 4:07 a.m., and you're thinking . . .

I'm awake. What's the time? The alarm goes off in only two more hours. If only I could go back to sleep. . . . Let's see. . . . What's the weather supposed to be? What should I wear? Do I have enough petrol in the car? I've got four new clients scheduled for this morning and then a consultation at the hospital later on. The next section of the book is due in a week. There goes the weekend. So much for catching up on lost sleep by sleeping late. I need to chase up Mum's house insurance claim – that means phoning the broker and getting stuck in the multiple-choice answering system forever. Better make sure that Trevor posted his college applications; the deadline's almost here. I've got to fill out all that financial stuff too. The boiler engineer never turned up yesterday – must remember to chase them for another appointment and book another day off. How much leave do I have left? I wonder whether I can fit in the gym tonight. Did I remember to take out the chicken for dinner? I really must stop thinking about all this . . . I need to go back to sleep. Okay, I'll try to concentrate on my breathing. Breathe in to the count of eight and then let it out slowly and then in . . .

Have you ever experienced early morning worry? As if falling asleep isn't hard enough, many people wake up before they want to, driven into high alert with anxious thoughts racing through their consciousness. In this chapter, you can find out how to get the best rest possible. Also, we show that what you do in the hours before going to bed can either help or hinder your sleep. Finally, you will see how to get rid of those recurrent nightmares once and for all.

The tendency towards early morning wakening with an inability to get back to sleep can be a sign of depression as well as anxiety. If your appetite changes, your energy decreases, your mood drops, your ability to concentrate diminishes, and you've lost interest in activities that you once found pleasurable, you may be clinically depressed. You should check with a mental health practitioner or a doctor to find out whether this is the case.

Giving Sleeplessness a Name

People generally need about eight hours of sleep per night. However, ask the average person how much they need, and they'll normally reply 'Five minutes more!' Older people may need a little less sleep, but this idea remains controversial among scientists. Besides, the real gauge as to whether you're getting enough sleep is how you feel during the daytime, not the exact number of hours you get. The Earth moves in a 24-hour cycle and so do we. Our body clocks synchronise us to our environment and even to the seasons' changing day lengths. For this we can thank *circadian rhythms* – programmes of around 24 hours (hence *circadian*, from the Latin *circa diem*, 'about a day') found in virtually all living things. Their most obvious signature is our sleep–wake cycles. Given that you are reading this book – hopefully not at 3 a.m. – you may well have discovered for yourself that anxiety frequently disrupts sleep, and a lack of sleep can increase your anxiety. The following list describes the most common sleep disturbances:

- **Disruption of circadian rhythm** occurs when your biological sleep clock is different from your actual sleep schedule. This condition happens when people work rotating shifts or travel across time zones.

- **Hormonal factors** may also play a part. Pregnant or menopausal women may suffer sleep disturbances. Hormonal fluctuations that occur during pregnancy and the menopause can cause physical discomfort and changes in body temperature that interrupt sleep.

- **Insomnia,** by far the most common sleep problem, may be the result of anxiety, depression, stress, poor sleep habits, discomfort, or an inadequate sleeping environment, such as a noisy block of flats or a lumpy mattress. Insomniacs have difficulty falling asleep and/or staying asleep.

- **Narcolepsy** occurs in the daytime rather than at night. It is a serious condition in which the person experiences sudden lapses of consciousness, falling asleep without warning, or experiences overwhelming feelings of sleepiness. Medication can help.

- **Nightmares** may increase with stress and anxiety. Of course, sometimes they just happen. In either event, if you suffer these frequently, they can disrupt the quality of your sleep. You may be afraid to try and go back to sleep, fearing that the nightmare will be waiting for you.

✔ **Decreased dreaming – dreamless sleep –** is less restful sleep. Scientists call the state of dreaming *rapid eye movement* (REM) sleep. During this time, the eyes shift rapidly and dreams occur. Interrupted sleep, certain drugs, and alcohol can interfere with getting enough REM sleep.

✔ **Prostate problems** may be disturbing enough to keep a man awake. Men who have an enlarged prostate gland may wake up numerous times during the night to urinate. If you wake up more than once a night to urinate, you may want to consult your doctor.

✔ **Restless leg syndrome,** more common among middle aged and older adults, produces the urge to keep moving because of uncomfortable feelings in the legs and feet. Certain prescription medication can help, so consult your doctor if you believe that you may suffer from this problem.

✔ **Snoring** sometimes indicates a more serious problem known as *sleep apnoea.* People with sleep apnoea actually stop breathing for short periods and wake up briefly to take a breath. Your partner snoring can also keep you awake.

Sleep apnoea can be a serious problem. If you or your partner snores heavily, you may want to consult a doctor or a sleep clinic. Many major hospitals have special clinics where your sleep can be monitored and assessed. Usually, you go there and spend the night in the sleep lab. Your family doctor can refer you to one of these specialised centres.

Sleep terror in children

Childhood sleep disorders, one of the most common complaints brought to pediatricians, can disrupt the whole family. Children usually outgrow many sleep disorders, such as bedwetting, frequent awakenings, and problems going to sleep, within a reasonable period.

Sleep terror, also know as night terror, is especially strange and frightening to many parents. It's relatively common, occurring among 1 to 6 per cent of all kids, but the incidence among adults is less than 1 per cent. Sleep terror tends to present itself about an hour and a half after going to bed. The child typically sits up suddenly and screams for up to half an hour. During the episode, the child is actually asleep and is difficult to awaken and comfort. Children don't remember their sleep terrors in the morning.

Sleep terror most often occurs when children are between the ages of four and ten. By the time a child is a teenager, the problem usually disappears.

Direct treatments for sleep terror are unavailable as yet. But then again, because children don't remember it, sleep terror usually doesn't cause the children who have it any daytime distress. Too little sleep may increase the likelihood of sleep terror, so parents should make sure that their children get enough sleep. And stress may also contribute to sleep terror, so parents should attempt to alleviate stress and other anxieties in their children. (See Chapter 17 for more information about how to help your kids cope with stress and anxiety.)

As you can see, much sleeplessness has a physical basis. At the same time, if your sleep is disrupted for any reason, and you have problems with anxiety, returning to sleep is more difficult. Obviously, you should explore the possible physical basis of any sleep problems. However, after you have done what you can with physical causes, you may still need to work on improving your sleep patterns.

The ABC of Getting Your Zs

Your sleep environment matters. Of course, some rare birds can sleep almost anywhere – on the couch, in a chair, on the floor, in the car, or even at their desks at work. On the other hand, most of us require the comfort of a bed and the right conditions. Sleep experts report that for a restful sleep, you should sleep in a room that's:

- ✔ **Dark:** You have a clock in your brain that tells you when it's time to sleep. Darkness helps set the clock by causing the brain to release melatonin, a hormone that helps to induce sleep. Consider putting up curtains that block out most of the sun if you find yourself awakened by the early morning light or if you need to sleep during the day. Some people even wear an eye mask to keep light out.

- ✔ **Cool:** People sleep better in a cool room. If you feel cold, adding blankets is usually preferable to a warm room.

- ✔ **Quiet:** If you live near a busy street or have loud neighbours, consider getting a fan or white-noise generator to block out nuisance noises. The worst kind of noise is intermittent and unpredictable. The various kinds of sporadic noise that can be blocked out by the sonsistent noise of a simple electric fan may amaze you.

- ✔ **Complete with a comfortable bed:** Mattresses matter. If you share your bed with another person or a pet, ensure that there's enough room for all of you.

In other words, make your bedroom a retreat that looks inviting and cosy. Spoil yourself with quality sheets and pillowcases. You may want to try aromatherapy (see Chapter 12 for more information). Many people claim that the fragrance of lavender helps them sleep, although no-one knows for sure whether it works.

Following a Few Relaxing Routines

Sleep revitalises your physical and mental resources. Studies show that sleep deprivation causes people to drive as if they are under the influence of alcohol.

Without sufficient sleep over long periods, people are likely to make more errors. Sleep deprivation makes you irritable, crabby, anxious, and despondent.

You need to schedule a reasonable amount of time for sleep – at least seven or eight hours. Don't burn the candle at both ends. We don't care how much work you have on your plate; depriving yourself of sleep can only make you less productive and less pleasant to be around.

So, first and foremost, allow sufficient time for sleep. But that's not enough if you have trouble with sleep, so we suggest that you look at the ideas in the subsections that follow to improve the quality of your sleep.

Associating sleep with your bed

One of the most important principles of sleep is to teach your brain to associate sleep with your bed. That means that when you get into bed, don't bring work along with you. Some people find that reading in bed relaxes them, and others like to watch a little TV before bed. That's fine if it works for you, but if those activities don't relax you, avoid doing them in bed.

If you go to bed and lie there for more than 20 or 30 minutes, unable to fall asleep, get up. Again, the point is to train your brain to link your bed to sleep. You can train your brain to dislike getting up by doing some unpleasant (though fairly passive, even boring) chore while you're awake. If you do this a number of times, your brain will find it easier to start feeling drowsy when you're in bed.

Just before hitting the sack

Some people find that taking a warm bath with fragrant oils or bath salts about an hour before hitting the hay is soothing. You may discover that soaking in a scented bath, in a dimly lit bathroom, while listening to relaxing music before going to bed is just the right ticket to solid slumber. Other people find one of the relaxation techniques discussed in Chapters 12 and 13 quite helpful. Studies show that relaxation can improve sleep.

Whenever possible, go to bed at close to the same time every night. Many people like to stay up late at weekends, and that's fine if you're not having sleep problems. But if you are, we recommend sticking to the same schedule as during the week. You need a regular routine and passive activities before bed.

Don't do strenuous physical or mental exercise within the few hours before going to sleep. Almost any stimulating activity can interfere with sleep.

Watching what you eat and drink

Obviously, you don't want to drink quantities of caffeinated drinks in the couple of hours before you go to bed. Don't forget that many sources other than coffee – colas, certain teas, chocolate, and certain pain relievers – contain caffeine. Of course, some people seem impervious to the effects of caffeine, while others are better off not consuming any after lunchtime. Even if you weren't bothered by caffeine in the past, you can develop sensitivity to it as you age. Consider caffeine's effects on you if you're having trouble sleeping.

Nicotine is also a stimulant. Try to avoid smoking just prior to bedtime. Obviously, it's preferable to quit smoking entirely, but if you haven't been able to stop yet, at least control how much you smoke before bedtime.

Alcohol relaxes the body and should be a great way of aiding sleep, but it isn't. That's because alcohol disrupts your sleep cycles. You don't get as much of the important REM sleep (discussed earlier in this chapter in the 'Giving Sleeplessness a Name' section), and you may find yourself waking during the night or up early in the morning, unable to get back to sleep. However, some people find that drinking a glass or two of wine in the evening is relaxing. That's fine, but watch the amount.

Heavy meals prior to going to bed aren't such a great idea either; many people find that eating too much before bed causes mild discomfort. In addition, you may want to avoid highly spiced and/or fatty foods prior to bed. However, going to bed hungry is also not a good idea; the key is balance.

So what should you eat or drink before bed? Herbal teas, such as chamomile or valerian, have many advocates. We don't have much data on how well they work, but herbal teas are quite unlikely to interfere with sleep, and they're pleasant to drink. Some evidence supports eating a small carbohydrate snack before bedtime to help induce sleep.

Medication options

Some people try treating their sleep problems with over-the-counter medications, many of which contain antihistamines that do help, but can lead to drowsiness the next day. Occasional use of these medications is relatively safe for most. Herbal formulas, such those containing valerian, may also help. (See Chapter 14 for more information on herbs.)

If sleep problems are chronic, you should consult your doctor. A medication that you're already taking may possibly be interfering with your sleep. Your doctor may prescribe medication to help induce sleep. Many sleep medications become less effective over time, and some carry the risk of addiction. These potentially addictive medications are only used for a short period. On the other hand, a few sleep medications work for a longer time as an aid to sleep without danger of addiction. Talk about your sleep problem with your doctor for more information and help.

What to Do When Sleep Just Won't Come

Becky sighs, realising that it's 2 a.m. and she has yet to fall asleep. She turns over and tries to be still, so that she doesn't wake her husband. She thinks, 'With everything I have to do tomorrow, if I don't sleep, I'll be a wreck. I hate not sleeping.' She gets out of bed, goes into the bathroom, finds the bottle of sleeping tablets, and pops three into her mouth. She's been taking them routinely for months, and they just don't seem to have the same effect that they did before.

She goes back to bed, tries to settle down, and worries about the bags under her eyes and what people will think. Her itchy dry skin starts to crawl. She can't stand the feeling of lying in bed for an eternity without sleeping.

In Becky's mind, her lack of sleep turns into a catastrophe, and all those thoughts about it actually makes it far more difficult for her to fall asleep. When you can't sleep, try to decatastrophise your problem by

- ✔ **Reminding yourself that every single time that you failed to sleep in the past, somehow you got through the next day in spite of your lack of sleep the night before.** The next day may not have been wonderful, but you survived.

- ✔ **Realising that occasional sleep loss happens to everyone.** Excessive worry can only aggravate the problem.

- ✔ **Getting up and distracting yourself with something else to do.** This stops your mind from magnifying the problem and can also prevent you from associating your bed with not sleeping.

- ✔ **Concentrating solely on your breathing.** See Chapter 16 for ideas on mindfulness and staying in the present moment as opposed to focusing on thoughts about the negative effects of your sleeplessness.

Many people try taking daytime naps when they consistently fail to sleep at night. It sounds like a great solution, but unfortunately it only compounds the problem. Frequent or prolonged naps disrupt your body's natural clock. If you must nap, make it a short, power nap, no longer than 20 minutes.

Of course, a few unusual people find that they can nap for just three or four minutes whenever they want during the day; they wake up refreshed and sleep well at night. If that's you, go ahead and nap. Most people simply can't do that.

Nagging Nightmares

Bad dreams plague almost everyone from time to time. However, some people find that nightmares invade their sleep on a nightly basis. Those who suffer from post-traumatic stress disorder (PTSD) are particularly likely to experience nightmares frequently. (For more information on PTSD, see Chapter 2.) Many people find nightmares emotionally upsetting, and these visions of horror can cause you to awaken and then wrestle with getting back to sleep.

A British clinical psychologist, Derek Jehu, and American psychiatrists Barry Krakow and Joseph Neidhardt have developed an effective strategy for getting rid of nightmares. You no longer have to feel like a helpless victim to these melodramas in your mind. Instead, you can take action to rid yourself of nightmares once and for all. Those suffering from PTSD may experience the same nightmare night after night. Others suffer nightmares involving new dramas of horror far more often than they want. Your nightmares may be repetitive or ever changing. Either way, you can use this technique:

1. **Develop your imagination.**

   Practise imagining and describing vivid scenes, just so long as they're pleasant and involve multiple senses. Do this when you're lying in bed with your eyes closed. Often people drop off to sleep in the middle of this exercise. And even if you don't – well, you had a great time on that gorgeous beach in Greece! You can also check Chapter 13 for more ideas on developing your imagination.

2. **Record your nightmares.**

   Keep a pad of paper and a pen at your bedside. When you wake from a nightmare, or first thing in the morning, write down as much as you can possibly conjure up about your nightmare. Be sure to write in the present tense and first person, for example 'I'm walking down this long, rocky road when . . . Describe the imagery with all your senses if you can. Leave some space on the page to write down any thoughts or memories that you associate with the nightmare.

   For example, **Vic** drives lorries for a living. A few years ago, he drove through a fog-filled stretch of motorway. Suddenly, without warning, he saw brake lights in front of him. He slammed on his brakes but couldn't stop in time. No sooner had he hit the lorry in front of him than he felt the impact of another vehicle slamming into his rear end. He heard horns blaring, metal crunching, and people screaming out from the foggy, surreal scene. Although terribly shaken, Vic sustained only minor cuts and bruises. Others in the 40-vehicle pile-up weren't so lucky.

Since that time, nightmares have plagued Vic almost nightly. He wakes up in a sweat and often spends the rest of the night sleepless. He records the following:

> I'm in my lorry driving somewhere, but I don't know where. My brakes give out, and I start gaining speed going downhill. I can smell the burning brake lining. I see cars start flying off the road in front of me for no reason. Then I see the old car my parents used to drive just ahead. Somehow I know they're in there. My mother's face appears in the rear window. At first she's laughing, but then her face turns to horror. I know I'm going to run into them. I can't stop.

Now he writes his thoughts and memories conjured up by the dream.

> I know that the brakes failing must be about the accident and the total lack of control that I felt. I also feel horribly guilty when I wake. Maybe that's about all the people who got hurt in the multiple pile-up that day. I especially think about the two kids who were killed. I wonder about the car with my parents. I remember learning how to drive in that car. So why would that be in my dream? Maybe it's because I started to feel that I wasn't that good a driver after the accident. But why are my parents in the dream, and why do I feel so guilty? I never really hurt them, or maybe I did. I still feel a little guilty about leaving Scotland for that job in Kent when they were getting on in years and didn't want me to go.

3. **Take the dream that bothers you and change the ending.**

This is the final step towards ridding yourself of nightmares: Create an ending that makes you feel better and puts you more in control; then imagine the new dream in vivid detail over and over again.

Read Vic's new, revised dream as follows:

> I'm in my lorry driving somewhere, but I don't know where. My brakes fail, and I start gaining speed going downhill. I hear the grinding as I force the lorry into a lower gear to slow it down. I see my parents' old car in front of me and an uphill turnoff just ahead. I know that I can steer my lorry right up into the turn off and come to a stop. I make the turn, and the truck stops. My parents see what's happened and turn around to follow me. We get out and hug.

Does something this simple work? Yes. Jehu's research has shown very positive results. Krakow and Neidhardt collaborated on a study and found that revising nightmares in this manner alleviated nightmare frequency and intensity for 70 per cent of the study's participants. This result lasted even after a year and a half had passed. Try it and sleep well.

Part IV
Focusing on Feeling

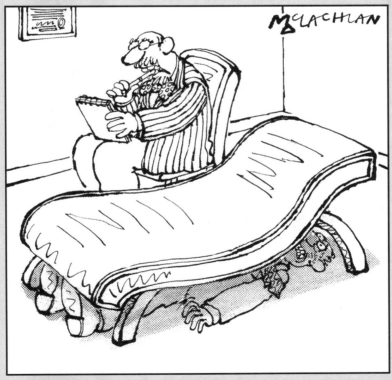

'Well, just to come here at all is a start
to curing your anxiety complex, Mr Gumbottle.'

In this part . . .

We point out that you can't feel anxious and relaxed at the same time. So we give you some quick, easy relaxation techniques for calming your mind and body. Address all your senses through breathing, muscle relaxation, aromatherapy, music, massage, and imagery.

Sometimes, you need a little more help to calm your anxiety. We review the various herbs and supplements that have been widely touted as anxiety cures. You'll see which ones work and which don't. We then help you decide if prescription medication looks like an approach for you to consider. You find out about the most commonly prescribed medications for anxiety – how they work, and their most frequent side effects.

Finally, we offer you a guide for letting go of anxiety through *acceptance*. You'll see that acceptance involves finding out how to let go of ego, tolerate uncertainty, embrace imperfection, and learn how to experience the present moment.

Chapter 12

Relaxation: The Five-Minute Solution

I don't have time to do anything of the fun, enjoyable things that I used to love. All my hobbies have fallen by the wayside. I seldom even relax. My life is far too hectic. I barely see my friends as it is now. I can't remember the last time I took a whole weekend off. I even neglect my own family. By the time I've cleared up after dinner, I'm so shattered I can't think about anything else. Usually I crawl off to bed, except when I collapse in front of the TV, and invariably within a few minutes I'm snoring, much to the family's annoyance. So much for quality relaxation there!'

Does this sound like you or someone you care about? When considering making lifestyle changes, the most frequent obstacle people put forward is that they don't have enough time to do all that they have to do, let alone want to do. Modern life moves at an ever-increasing pace. Pagers and mobiles pursue you from work to home, in the car, when you're out for the evening, and sometimes even when you retire to bed.

We asked a wise Yogi how long he practises every day, fully expecting to hear the discouraging answer, 'An hour or two.' Imagine our surprise when he told us, 'Five minutes.' That's all he needs. He went on to explain that he usually takes more time, but he only commits to five minutes out of each day.

Realistically, five minutes isn't a great deal of time. Everyone can find five minutes. And if you do five minutes, it just may stretch into 10 or 20. But if it doesn't, that really is okay. Relaxation slowly permeates your life without you even knowing it, and when anxiety hits, you'll have a valuable tool for calming the storm within.

In this chapter, the relaxation procedures fall into one of three major categories: breathing techniques, ways for relaxing the body, and sensory experiences. Some of these can take a little longer to become good at, but they can all be done in five minutes when you get the hang of them. The key is daily practice. Like every other skill, the more you practise, the easier and faster it gets.

Blowing Anxiety Away

Breathing is something you've practised more than anything else in your life. In waking moments, you don't normally even think about your breathing. And it's a safe bet to say that most of us aren't aware of thinking about breathing while we are asleep either. Yet, of all our biological functions, breathing is the most critical to life. Without oxygen, we die! You can go weeks without food, and a couple of days without water, but only minutes without breathing at all. You need oxygen to purify the bloodstream, burn up waste products, and rejuvenate every part of the body and mind. If you're not getting enough oxygen, then your

✔ Thinking becomes sluggish

✔ Blood pressure goes up

✔ Heart rate increases

You'll also get dizzy, shaky, and depressed.

Many people react to stress with rapid, shallow breathing that messes up the optimum ratio of oxygen to carbon dioxide in the blood. This phenomenon is called *hyperventilation,* and it causes a variety of distressing symptoms:

✔ Blurred vision

✔ Disorientation

✔ Jitteriness

✔ Loss of consciousness

✔ Muscle cramps

✔ Poor concentration

✔ Rapid pulse

✔ Tingling sensations in the extremities or face

Anxiety and relaxation: A recipe for incompatibility

Have you ever known two people who couldn't be in the same room at the same time? If they show up at the same party, there's bound to be trouble. They're like oil and water – they just don't mix.

Anxiety and relaxation are a little like that. Think about it. How can you be anxious at the same time that you're relaxed? Not an easy accomplishment. Psychologists have a term for this phenomenon – *reciprocal inhibition*. Many psychologists believe that the techniques described in this chapter work because relaxation inhibits anxiety and anxiety inhibits relaxation. Training yourself in the use of relaxation skills should therefore help you inhibit your anxiety.

Hyperventilation frequently accompanies panic attacks as well as chronic anxiety. Many of the symptoms of over-breathing feel like symptoms of anxiety, and many people with anxiety disorders tend to hyperventilate. Therefore, finding out how to breathe properly is considered to be an effective antidote to anxiety.

When you came into the world, unless you had a physical problem with your lungs, you probably had no problems breathing – in fact, after you started, you just didn't stop. Look at most babies. Unless they're in distress from hunger, thirst, pain, or cold, they need no instruction on how to breathe in a slow, even, regular way, or in how to relax. Their little tummies rise and fall with each breath in a rhythmic, natural way. The stresses of everyday life, however, can mess up your inborn, natural breathing response.

Under stress, breathing often becomes shallow and fast. People sometimes hold their breath when they feel stressed and aren't even aware of doing it. Try noticing your breathing when you feel stressed and see whether you're a breath-holder or a rapid, shallow breather.

You can also see what your breathing is like when you're not stressed:

1. **Lie down on your back.**

2. **Put one hand on your stomach and the other on your chest.**

3. **Notice the movements of your hands as you breathe.**

   If you're breathing correctly, the hand on your stomach rises as you inhale and lowers as you exhale. The hand on your chest doesn't move so much, and to the extent that it does, it should do so in tandem with the other hand.

The odds are that if you have a problem with anxiety, your breathing probably needs some attention. That's especially so if you have trouble with panic attacks, which we discuss in Chapter 2. Breathing practice can start you on the way towards feeling calmer.

The benefits of controlled breathing

Just in case you think that improving the way you breathe sounds like a rather unimaginative, simplistic way to reduce anxiety, you may want to consider the healthy effects. Studies show that training in breathing can contribute to the reduction of panic attacks within a matter of a few weeks. Other studies have indicated that as well as calming worry, controlled breathing can slightly reduce blood pressure, improve the heart's rhythm, reduce certain types of epileptic seizures, sharpen mental performance, increase blood circulation, and possibly even improve the outcome of cardiac rehabilitation efforts following a heart attack. Not a bad list of benefits for such a simple skill.

Abdominal breathing for only five minutes a day

Figure out how to breathe with your *diaphragm*. This is the muscle that lies between your abdominal cavity and your lung cavity. Try this exercise to start breathing like a baby again. You may want to lie down, or you can do this while sitting if you have a large comfortable chair in which you can stretch out.

1. **Check your body for tension. Notice whether certain muscles feel tight or whether your breathing is shallow and rapid. See whether you're clenching your teeth or whether you have other distressing feelings.**

   You may rate your tension on a scale from 1 to 10, with 1 representing complete relaxation and 10 meaning total tension.

2. **Place a hand on your stomach.**

3. **Breathe in slowly through your nose and fill the lower part of your lungs.**

   You'll know you're doing this correctly if your hand rises from your abdomen.

4. **Pause and hold your breath for a moment.**

5. **Exhale slowly.**

   As the air goes out, imagine that your entire body is deflating like a balloon and let it go limp.

6. **Pause briefly again.**

7. **Inhale the same way slowly through your nose to a slow count of four.**

   Check to see that your hand rises from your abdomen. Your chest should move only slightly and in tandem with your stomach.

8. **Pause and hold your breath briefly.**

9. **Exhale to a slow count of six.**

   At first, if you find that hard to do, use a count of four. Later, you'll find that slowing down to a count of six is easier.

10. **Continue breathing in and out in this fashion for five minutes.**

11. **Check your body again for tension and rate that tension on a scale of 1 to 10.**

We recommend that you do this exercise once a day for five minutes. You'll find it relaxing, and it won't add stress to your day by taking up much of your valuable time. Try it for five minutes for ten days in a row. After you do that, try noticing your breathing at various times during your regular routine. You'll quickly see whether you're breathing through the diaphragm, or through the upper chest like so many people do. Slowly but surely, abdominal breathing can become a new habit that decreases your stress.

Breathing by the book

Okay, just in case you're having trouble getting the hang of abdominal breathing, we have another way to help you discover the skill. You'll need a book – this one will do fine. This technique may seem strange, but you'll find it easy to do.

1. **Check over your body for tension and rate the tension on a scale from 1 to 10, with 1 representing complete relaxation and 10 being total tension.**

2. **Read through steps 3 to 12. Remember them? Then off you go.**

3. **Open this book to approximately the centre.**

4. **Lie down on your back on a bed, a couch, or the floor.**

5. **Place the open book on your stomach with the open pages on your stomach and the binding facing away from your stomach.**

6. **Take a moment to simply relax.**

7. **Inhale slowly through your nose so that the book rises.**

8. **Hold your breath briefly and exhale slowly.**

9. **Continue breathing this way. Allow your breathing to be slow, easy, and regular.**

10. **Inhale and allow the book to rise; then exhale and watch the book slowly drop.**

11. **Continue breathing this way for five minutes: Notice the feelings in your body as you do. Pay attention to how the air feels going in your nostrils, into your lungs, and out again.**

12. **Rate the tension in your body again on a scale from 1 to 10.**

All it takes is five minutes a day of breathing practice; everyone can find five minutes.

After you've practised book or abdominal breathing for ten days, notice your breathing throughout the day. Allow your diaphragm to develop the habit of taking charge of your breathing. You'll feel better a little at a time.

Whenever you feel anxiety or panic coming on, try using one of these breathing exercises. You may head anxiety or panic off at the pass. On the other hand, anxiety and especially panic may rise to a level that makes these exercises more difficult. If that happens to you, try our panic-breathing technique.

Panic breathing

Occasionally you may need a faster, more powerful technique. Perhaps you're at a shopping centre and feel trapped, or maybe you're on your way to a job interview and feel overwhelmed. Whatever the situation, when stress hits you and it feels like an unexpected punch in the stomach, try our panic-breathing technique.

1. **Inhale deeply and slowly through your nose.**

2. **Hold your breath for a slow count of six.**

3. **Slowly breathe out through your lips to a count of eight, making a slight hissing sound as you do.**

   That sound can be so soft that only you can hear it. You don't have to worry about what anyone around you may think.

4. **Repeat the above between five to ten times.**

You may think that panic breathing will be difficult to do when stress suddenly strikes like a lightning bolt. We won't deny it takes some practice. However, children have successfully discovered how to use this technique when they face painful medical procedures. When the children used the panic-breathing technique, they felt a little calmer and reported feeling less distress and pain. The key is the slight hissing sound, which gives you a much easier way to slow down your breath.

If panic breathing doesn't help, and you feel like you may be having a full-blown panic attack that won't go away, try breathing in and out of a paper bag. If you are hyperventilating, as people often do during a panic attack, the air that you breathe out is very rich in carbon dioxide, and so the level of carbon dioxide in the blood drops lower and lower. As the level of carbon dioxide decreases and the amount of oxygen in the blood increases, your body releases a variety of chemicals that put you in a state of high alert. See Chapter 2 for more on stress, anxiety, and the fight or flight response. You feel a whole host of the physical symptoms of anxiety (racing heart, sweating, and so on), and it's pretty uncomfortable. Breathing into the bag lets you re-inhale some of the carbon-dioxide-rich air that you have just exhaled and so rebalances the ratio of oxygen to carbon dioxide, which should cut the panic attack short.

Mantra breathing

Mantras are often used for various types of meditation. For some people, a mantra is a word with some type of spiritual connotation. One of the off-shoots of the Hindu religion purportedly first developed the use of a mantra to be used by a Guru in a ceremony. The mantra was said to have special powers that could result in redemption.

Mantras have also been chanted as a non-religious technique, much as we suggest in this chapter. They've been employed to modulate breathing in addition to their use with meditation. Using a mantra to relax your breathing is surprisingly easy.

1. **Choose a meaningless word or a string of letters that has a pleasing, smooth sound.** Although the word may have no particular meaning, if it is suggestive of relaxation, all the better. You can use any word you want. You can also pick something neutral, such as *one,* or a word with a meaning that actually relates to relaxation, such as *relax, calm,* or *peace.* Some people even use a short phrase, such as 'let go . . . relax' or 'calming . . . down'. Examples of meaningless words or sounds are

   mmmmmmm

   iiimmmmmm

   aiiinnnnnnng

   ohhmmmmmm

   shiiiiiiammm

   shaaaammmm

   shalooommm

2. **Find a comfortable place to sit.**

3. **Close your eyes.**

4. **Slowly begin repeating your mantra out loud. Stretch one full pronunciation out to about ten seconds.**

5. **Gradually allow your voice to get lower and lower as you say your mantra.**

6. **If thoughts come up, just notice them and then focus back on repeating your mantra.**

7. **Continue for 15 to 20 minutes.**

Hang on a second – we promised five minutes! Five minutes will do, it really will. But do try it for a little longer at first. Later, you can shorten it to five minutes and do it at any time that you want. If you really only have five minutes, then you can do it for just five minutes from day one. Any length of time is useful. Sometimes, you may want to continue longer; at other times, that won't be the case, and that's okay.

The gentle inhale/exhale technique

You're likely to find that the gentle inhale/exhale breathing technique is the simplest of all the exercises. It takes just a few minutes and requires only a small amount of attention.

1. **Find a comfortable place to sit down.**

2. **Notice your breathing: Feel the air as it flows through your nostrils and into your lungs. Feel your muscles pull the air in and push it out.**

3. **Let your breathing flow rhythmically, evenly, and smoothly.**

4. **Imagine that you're holding a flower with dainty, delicate petals up to your nose. Allow your breath to soften so that the petals remain undisturbed.**

5. **Rhythmically breathe in and out with an even flow.**

6. **Continue to notice the air as it passes through your airways.**

7. **Notice how focusing on nothing but your breathing gently relaxes your mind and body.**

8. **Allow the air to refresh you.**

9. **Continue your gentle breathing and just focus solely on all the sensations of smooth, even breathing.**

Work on the gentle inhale/exhale technique for five minutes a day for ten days. You may then find that you want to continue with one or more of our breathing techniques each day of your life. After all, you have to breathe anyway, so you may as well do it in a relaxing, anxiety-reducing manner.

Chilling Out

Some of you may find that breathing techniques quickly calm your anxiety. Others may require a technique that concentrates on total-body relaxation. Researchers have discovered a whole host of benefits from body relaxation training methods. These are now included in the vast majority of anxiety treatment programmes. We describe three types of body relaxation: progressive muscle, autogenic, and applied relaxation.

Relaxing by tightening: Progressive muscle relaxation

Over half a century ago, Edmund Jacobsen developed what came to be the most widely used relaxation technique, *progressive muscle relaxation*. You can find a wide variety of similar techniques, all described as progressive muscle relaxation, in various books and journals. Each of them may use slightly different muscle groups or go through the muscle groups in a different order, but they all do essentially the same thing.

Progressive muscle relaxation involves going through various muscle groups in the body and tensing each one for a little while, followed by a quick letting go of the tension. You then pay close attention to the sensation of release, noticing how the limp muscles feel in contrast to their previous tense state.

Getting ready to mellow

You'll find it useful to look for the right place in which to do your progressive muscle relaxation. You probably don't have a soundproof room, but find the quietest place that you can. Consider unplugging the phone and turning off your mobile.

Choose some comfortable clothing or loosen any clothing you are wearing that's tight and constricting. Take off your shoes, belt, or anything that's uncomfortable.

Realise that when you begin tensing each muscle group, you shouldn't over-exert; don't tighten using more than about two-thirds of your strongest effort. You want firm tension, but you're not body building. When you tense, hold the tension for six to ten seconds and notice how it feels. Then let go of the tension all at once, as though a string holding the muscles up has been cut.

After you release the muscles, focus on the relaxed feeling and allow it to deepen for 10 to 15 seconds. If you don't achieve the desired state of relaxation for that muscle group, you can try once or twice more if you want.

Be aware that you can't *force* relaxation to happen. You *allow* it to happen. Perfectionists struggle with this idea. Don't force it and do try and banish the idea that you *must* do this exercise *perfectly*. Remember it's a skill that you'll acquire slowly over time.

When you tighten one muscle group, try to keep all the other muscles in your body relaxed. Doing this takes a little practice, but you can figure out how to tense one body area at a time. Try and make sure you keep your face relaxed when you're tensing any area other than your face. Yoga instructors often say, 'Soften your eyes.' Though it's unclear exactly what that means, this instruction has often been found helpful – whatever it is that you are actually doing to achieve it.

Occasionally, relaxation training makes people feel surprisingly uncomfortable. If this happens to you, simply stop. If it continues to occur with repeated practice, you may want to seek professional help. Also, don't tighten any part of your body that makes you feel uncomfortable. Avoid tightening any area that's suffered injury or has given you frequent trouble, such as your lower back.

Discovering the progressive muscle technique

Now you're ready to start. Sit down in your chosen place and get comfortable.

1. **Take a deep breath, hold it, concentrate on the feelings, and then let the tension go.**

   Pulling the air in from your abdomen, breathe deeply. (See the section 'Abdominal breathing for only five minutes a day', earlier in this chapter, if you're unclear about this.) Hold your breath for three or four seconds and slowly let the air out. Imagine your whole body is a balloon losing air as you exhale and let tension go out with the air. Take three more such breaths and feel your entire body getting more and more limp with each breath.

2. **Squeeze your hands tight and then relax.**

   Squeeze your fingers into a fist. Feel the tension and hold it for six to ten seconds. Then, all at once, release your hands and let them go limp. Allow the tension in your hands to flow out. Let the relaxation deepen for 10 to 15 seconds.

3. **Tighten your arms and then relax.**

Bend your lower arms up so your hands are against your shoulders, and tighten all the arm muscles. Make sure you tense the muscles on the inside and outside of both the upper and lower arms. If you're not sure whether you're doing that, use one hand to do a tension check on the other arm. Hold the tension a little while and then drop your arms as though you've cut the string holding them up. Let the tension flow out and the relaxation flow in.

4. **Raise up your shoulders, tighten, and then relax.**

Raise your shoulders up to your ears, as though you were a turtle trying to get its head back into its shell. Hold the tension and then let your shoulders drop. Feel the relaxation deepen for 10 to 15 seconds.

5. **Tighten and relax the muscles in your upper back.**

Pull your shoulders back and bring your shoulder blades closer together. Hold that tension a little while . . . and let it go.

6. **Scrunch up your entire face and then relax.**

Squeeze your forehead down, screw up your eyes, and furrow your eyebrows. Clench your jaws together and contract your tongue and lips. Let the tension grow and hold it . . . then relax and let go.

7. **Tighten and relax the back of your neck.**

Avoid causing yourself pain. Gently let your head tip backwards towards your back and feel the muscles tighten in the back of your neck. Notice that tension and hold it; let go and relax. Feel relaxation deepening.

8. **Contract the front neck muscles and then loosen them.**

Gently lower your chin towards your chest. Tighten your neck muscles and let the tension increase and maintain it; then relax. Feel the tension melting away like candle wax.

9. **Tighten the muscles in your stomach and chest and maintain the tension. Then let it go.**

Concentrate on noticing the difference between when the muscles are tense and when they are relaxed. Allow yourself to enjoy the sensations when your muscles relax.

10. **Arch your back, hang on to the contraction, and then relax.**

Be gentle with your lower back and skip this exercise entirely if you've ever had trouble with this part of your body. Tighten these muscles by arching your lower back, pressing your shoulders back against the chair, or tensing the muscles any way you want. Gently increase and maintain the tension, but not too much. Now relax and allow the waves of relaxation to roll in.

11. **Contract and relax the muscles in your buttocks.**

    Tighten your buttocks to gently lift yourself up in your chair. Hold the tension. Then let tension melt and relaxation grow.

12. **Squeeze and relax your thigh muscles.**

    Tighten and hold these muscles. Then relax and feel the tension draining out; let the calm deepen and spread.

13. **Contract and relax your calves.**

    Tighten the muscles in your calves by lifting the balls of your feet upwards while keeping your heels on the floor. Pull your toes upwards. Take care; if you ever get muscle cramps, don't overdo this exercise. Hold the tension . . . then let go. Let tension drain into the floor.

14. **Gently curl your toes downwards, maintain the tension, and then relax.**

    Again, focus on the differences you can feel. Let both of your feet go limp and floppy.

15. **Take a little time to scan your entire body.**

    Notice whether you feel different to when you began. If you find any areas of tension, allow the relaxed areas around them to come in and replace the tension with relaxation. If that doesn't work, repeat the tense-and-relax procedure for the tense area.

16. **Spend a few minutes enjoying the relaxed feelings.**

    Let relaxation spread and penetrate every muscle fibre in your body. Notice any feelings you have. You may feel warmth, or you may feel a floating sensation. Perhaps you'll feel a sense of sinking down. Whatever it is, allow it to happen. When you feel ready, you can open your eyes and carry on with your day, perhaps feeling like you just returned from a short holiday.

Some people like to make a recording of the progressive muscle relaxation instructions to make it easier to go through the exercises without referring to a book. If you do, be sure to record your instructions to yourself using a slow, calming tone of voice.

In the beginning, take a little longer than five minutes to go through the steps of progressive muscle relaxation. You'll find it most effective if you take 20 or 30 minutes to go through the exercises when you first start learning the technique. The more you practise, the more quickly you'll find that you can slide into serenity. So even if you listen to a recording, consider shortening the procedure on your own after a while. For example, you can tense all the muscles in your lower body at once, followed by all your upper body muscles. At other times, you may want to simply tense and relax a few body areas that carry most of your tension. Most frequently these are your neck, shoulder, and back muscles. Some people say that they eventually discover how to relax in just one minute when they've become proficient.

Extolling the virtues of progressive muscle relaxation

Many people believe that for a remedy to be truly effective, it must take plenty of work and possibly feel a little painful – the no pain, no gain philosophy. As you can see, progressive muscle relaxation isn't especially arduous, and it actually feels good, so can it really do anything for you? Well, for starters, progressive relaxation training is usually a component of most successful treatment programmes for anxiety.

However, studies also show that progressive muscle relaxation can effectively reduce various types of chronic pain, such as the pain associated with ulcerative colitis and cancer and headaches. It also works to reduce insomnia and may improve the functioning of your immune system. A study published in the December 2001 issue of the *Journal of Clinical Psychology* found that in addition to inducing greater relaxation, progressive muscle relaxation also led to increased mental quiet and joy.

Neuropsychological Rehabilitation (1999, Volume 9) reported that for patients with Alzheimer's disease, progressive muscle relaxation actually improved both their behavioural problems as well as their performance on verbal fluency and memory tasks. A 2003 study by Hull University reported encouraging results for using progressive muscle relaxation and hypnosis in addition to medical treatment for cancer. And research has also shown that people can learn applied muscle tension based on the tensing stage of progressive muscle relaxation, which can help stop them from fainting, for instance, at the sight of blood.

We aren't suggesting that progressive muscle relaxation cures Alzheimer's or cancer, whisks away all your pain, or eradicates all your anxiety. However, many studies clearly show that it exerts benefits across a surprisingly wide range of problems. We recommend that you give it a try.

Sizing up self-hypnosis: Autogenic training

Autogenic (meaning 'produced from one's self') training was introduced well over half a century ago, just a few years after Jacobson developed progressive muscle relaxation. Shulz, the German neuropsychiatrist who developed this strategy for reducing stress, based his technique on self-hypnosis and the power of suggestion.

Autogenic training is the most passive way of relaxing. All relaxation techniques work better if you approach them by allowing them to happen rather than forcing anything. However, autogenic training is actually based on not *doing* anything; it simply involves passive responses to suggestions. Other chapters discuss how thoughts can enormously increase your anxiety. Fortunately, the opposite is true as well. Calm ideas elicit a sense of relaxation almost as a reflex, if you let them.

Your mind automatically associates certain responses with different words and images. For example, imagine cutting a mango with a sharp knife and seeing the juice squirt out as you slice. Imagine picking up half the mango, smelling it, opening your mouth, and taking a large bite into the juicy, pulpy flesh of the mango. Now, back to reality. Are you salivating? If so, words alone created this response.

In fact, if you try to salivate without any words or images, you're likely to fail. You just can't make some responses happen. The same goes for relaxation. Try it and see. Imagine that you're hooked up to a machine that measures your tension levels by analysing your muscle tension, heart rate, and other physical responses to stress. Then we offer you a million pounds if you do nothing but relax. That's right; a million pounds. Oh, and by the way, to give you even more motivation, we hold a gun to your head and tell you that if you fail to relax, we'll fire the gun. Now RELAX! Do you think that you may just have some difficulty?

Realise that relaxation is accomplished by letting go. You allow it to happen as a natural response to calming suggestions. You can't force relaxation.

Autogenic relaxation involves thinking about your body and letting it go into a comfortable, calm state. Lie down, loosen your clothing or put on some more comfortable clothing, close your eyes, and spend time focusing on each of the autogenic concepts that follow, while you imagine that you feel heavy and warm, that your heart is quiet, and that your breathing is ever soooooo eeeeeeasy. Try focusing on each concept separately until you've seen what it can do for you. Then you can see what it feels like to combine them.

Just think about the words and images that autogenic training presents to you; don't try to make anything happen because, if you do, you'll sabotage the process. Hear the words over and over:

- ✔ **Heavy:** My hands, arms, and legs feel heavy . . . They are soooo heavy. I don't have to do anything at all because they're so heavy that I can't lift them if I want to. My hands and arms are heavy . . . very, very heavy. Gravity weighs down my arms and draws tension away. Tension is draining . . . heavy like weights are strapped around my arms . . . very heavy. My legs are heavy . . . very, very heavy. Weights strapped around my legs . . . sinking . . . relaxed and calm . . . sinking into a state of calm and serenity . . . do nothing and no need to make anything happen. Worries and concerns are melting away, sinking out of sight quietly and peacefully.

- ✔ **Warm:** My arms and legs are warm and heavy. A desert sun shines its rays on my arms and legs. It penetrates the skin and muscles . . . tension melting . . . warm and serene . . . warm blankets wrapped around me . . . I'm submersed in a warm whirlpool of circulating water, sinking into calm and relaxation . . . feeling tension float away . . . dissolving . . . warm, melting . . . no need to make anything happen. The sun warms my body, serene and placid . . . sinking . . . so warm and calm . . . peaceful and relaxed.

✔ **Quiet heart: Place one hand over your heart. Remind yourself that your heart is beating.** My heart beat is strong and steady, even and calm . . . nothing to do . . . so steady and strong . . . heart rhythmically thumping . . . like a steady, slow drum beat . . . sinking into a river of relaxation . . . tension fading . . . heart regular, strong, steady . . . steady, drumming, beating, relaxation deepening, soothing and quiet . . . a time to let worries go . . . warm, calm, steady . . . peaceful and relaxed.

✔ **Easy breathing: Sit in a comfortable position and remind yourself that your breathing is soooo rhythmic and eeeeasy.** I don't need to breathe in any particular way. Just let it happen. My body is finding its own breathing rhythm and pace. . . no worries; tension easing away; relaxed, even, calm, serene, easy, flowing breath. My body just takes over and breathes how it wants . . . peaceful . . . air flowing easily in and out . . . in and out . . . so calm and relaxed . . . smooth and effortless . . . steady and rhythmic.

Relaxing when it counts: Applied relaxation

Discovering how to relax using breathing techniques, progressive muscle relaxation, or autogenic training may help you reduce your anxiety. But if you just do these activities when you're lying in bed or spending a quiet day at home, you miss the opportunity to challenge your fears with a powerful tool. *Applied relaxation* means taking the techniques that you practised and putting them to work in the situations in which you're under the most stress.

The key to success lies in the mastery of the technique in non-stressful settings before taking the next step. For example, perhaps you've practised the progressive relaxation technique many times, and you can tighten and loosen your muscles to achieve a state of relaxation in just a few minutes.

Is autogenic training worthwhile?

Can something as passive and effortless as autogenic training really do anything for you? Actually, the studies on its effectiveness haven't all been as scientifically sound as the studies on progressive muscle relaxation. Nevertheless, autogenic training is a very popular type of relaxation training among European professionals. A number of reasonably sound studies suggest that it has stress-reducing value in addition to controlling various anxiety disorders, reducing motion sickness, and easing certain types of chronic muscle pain and the pain and distress that follow coronary bypass surgery. A study published in the journal *Complementary Therapies in Medicine* (2000, Volume 8) found that it's at least as effective as standard anti-anxiety medication for treating generalised anxiety disorder. (See Chapter 2 for a description of generalised anxiety disorder.)

Now that you've mastered the technique in a non-stressful setting, think of a particular situation that frightens you. A common one is public speaking. Perhaps you've agreed to speak at a large event with an audience of several hundred people. Prior to your speech, you practise your favourite relaxation technique. You try to maintain that state of relaxation as you walk up to give your speech, but you experience feelings of panic nonetheless. What happens?

That's pretty much what we would expect because applied relaxation works best if you break the tasks into smaller, more manageable steps. For example, you can practise relaxation while preparing a talk for a small audience. Then you can practise relaxation while thinking about giving your talk to the small group. Now repeat this process with a larger audience, so that you continue your practice in graduated, small steps. (Discover more about how to take small, graduated steps in Chapter 8.)

Relaxing Via Your Senses

Your path to finding relaxation may lead you through a variety of experiences. We can't possibly know which direction will work best for you. You have to experiment with various approaches to discover your own most effective relaxation remedies. In this section, we ask that you allow your senses to soothe you.

Sounds to soothe the savage beast

Ever since people populated the planet, they have turned to music for solace. From primitive drums to symphony orchestras, sound elicits emotion. The emotions are wide ranging, including patriotic fervour, love, excitement (sexual or otherwise), fear, and relaxation. The power of music is the basis of the whole profession of music therapy. Music therapists work in hospitals, schools, and nursing homes, using sounds to unlock emotions and memories, and to soothe distress.

But you don't need to be a music therapist to make use of music's power. You probably already know what types of music calm you. Perhaps you love classical music or jazz. You may not have thought of trying out a tape or CD of ocean waves, babbling brooks, whispering wind, birdsong, or other sounds of nature. Many find those sounds quite relaxing, and although it makes no sense to us, some teenagers say that they feel relaxed listening to heavy metal. Work that one out.

Visit any well-stocked music shop or Web site and explore a wide range of possibilities. Experiment and try new sounds. Many of these recordings say that they contain specially mixed music to maximise relaxation.

The applied advantage

Afraid of the dentist? *Applied relaxation* (applying a relaxation technique to a stressful situation) can help you deal with your fears. A Scandinavian study found that applied relaxation decreased the fear of a trip to the dentist and helped people to get the treatment that they needed but had been avoiding. Applied relaxation has also been used successfully to treat generalised anxiety disorder. Furthermore, this approach appears to help people with panic disorder. (See Chapter 2 for descriptions of generalised anxiety disorder and panic disorder.) One of the most common uses of applied relaxation is for relief from chronic pain.

Buyer beware! Don't buy just any recording that you see with the word *relaxation* on the label. Unfortunately, some are not very useful. Either get recommendations or listen to some recordings in the shop. On some Web sites, you can even listen to a sample before you buy your Internet purchase.

Only the nose knows for sure

Ever walked through a shopping centre and smelled freshly baked cinnamon rolls or freshly brewed coffee? Perhaps you were tempted to buy just because of the aroma. The temptation can be so powerful as to make you wonder whether those enticing aromas are no accident, but are deliberately pumped into the entire shopping centre ventilation system, just to tempt you!

In addition to making you hungry and thirsty, the scents may also trigger pleasant emotions and memories. Perhaps a scent took you back to an earlier enjoyable experience, all by itself, with no effort required by you.

A huge perfume industry exploits the power of aromas to attract and seduce. Manufacturers of deodorants, lotions, powders, hairsprays, and air fresheners also capitalise on the power of smell. We suggest that you can explore the ability of aromas to calm your jangled nerves.

Aromatherapy makes use of various essential oils – those natural substances extracted from plants. These substances are said to affect both physical and emotional health. We can't vouch for these claims because few good studies exist on their effects. But the theory behind aromatherapy seems to have some potential validity because the cranial nerve transmits messages from the nose into the parts of the brain that control mood, memories, and appetite.

One study reported in 2006 has suggested that aromatherapy is a useful treatment in mild or moderate insomnia. Although the active treatment effects are not strong, aromatherapy can be a useful alternative to prescribed sleeping tablets because there seems to be no morning hangover.

If you have a physical illness, please consult a qualified doctor because aromatherapy isn't likely to cure you. No-one knows whether aromatherapy truly promotes good health. Also don't use aromatherapy when pregnant, or allow children to use them.

However, if you want to experiment with various aromas to see whether any of them help you relax, go for it. Preliminary studies have suggested that certain aromas may reduce anxiety, decrease nicotine-withdrawal symptoms, and get rid of headaches. Lemon balm *(Melissa)* has a longstanding history in herbal medicine for treating insomnia and calming anxiety. Studies also suggest a positive effect on clarity of thinking and mood. So giving aromatherapy a try probably won't hurt.

Consider the following aromatherapy scent suggestions, but be sure to shop around because prices can vary substantially. A trusted local health food store may be a good place to start.

- Chamomile
- Eucalyptus
- Lavender
- Neroli *(Citrus aurantium)*
- Lemon balm *(Melissa officinalis)*

These essential oils may help relieve anxiety and combat sleeplessness. They do smell pretty good, so put a few drops in your warm bath or on your pillow. Have a good sleep.

Massaging away stress

Pets, particularly cats and dogs, often come to their owners and demand to be stroked, gently scratched, or petted. Not only does the pet enjoy it, but there have been studies suggesting that having the chance to stroke a pet on a regular basis improves the health and the mood of the person doing the stroking.

People need to be touched too. It's great to be hugged and stroked by the people we care about. Massage by a qualified professional can enable you to enjoy the sensation of being touched and also help you to relax. If you've never indulged, consider treating yourself to a massage. In years past, only the elite sought massage therapy. Today, people flock to massage therapists to reduce stress, manage pain, and just to feel good.

Everybody needs touching

In the 1940s, many European babies ended up in orphanages. A shocking number of these orphans failed to grow or interact with others, and some appeared to fade away and die for no discernible reason. They had sufficient food, clothing, and shelter. A physician named Dr Spitz investigated and found that the orphans' failure to thrive appeared to be due to a lack of human touch. In other words, the care-givers provided nutrients but not contact.

At the 2005 British Psychological Society Conference, Anna Cheshire and colleagues at Coventry University revealed that teaching parents of children with cerebral palsy how to massage their children led to a significant increase in the children's satisfaction with life. The parents also thought it improved their children's sleeping, mobility, and verbal communication.

In the US, psychologist Tiffany Field and her colleagues found that premature infants who were given regular massages gained more weight than those who merely received standard medical care. Other studies by this research group have included normal babies as well as infants born with HIV or cocaine addiction and young children with diabetes, eating disorders, or asthma. Babies and children who receive a massage regularly have lower amounts of stress hormones and lower levels of anxiety than those who don't. Other benefits that were identified include pain reduction, increased attentiveness, and enhanced immune function.

If it's this good for babies, we reckon that it's pretty good for you. And it's not just the person receiving the massage who benefits: A 2006 study showed that mothers massaging their babies reduces anxiety and depression – in the mothers. So indulge!

Other than your partner, you should only go to a qualified masseur or masseuse. Massage therapy is *not* a sexual encounter, although some in the sex trade masquerade as massage therapists in so-called massage parlours.

Although long considered an alternative medical intervention with dubious value, new research has fuelled interest in the benefits of massage. A study published in 2001 in the *International Journal of Neuroscience* found that massage increased work productivity and reduced work-related injuries.

Another way of getting a massage is to sit in a whirlpool for five minutes. This can be really relaxing because, in addition to the massage that you get from the force of the water jets, the feel of the warm water that's forced into the whirlpool and the sound of the water rushing around – like ocean waves rolling onto the beach – also has a calming effect. Although some homes have whirlpools built into their baths, most health spas and gyms also have whirlpools that people can enjoy for a small fee in excess of the basic membership.

Chapter 13

Creating Calm in Your Imagination

· ·

In This Chapter

▶ Honing the powers of your imagination

▶ Imagining your way to relaxation

▶ Developing your powers of observation

▶ Creating your own images

· ·

*P*eople who have vivid imaginations (perhaps people like you) can think themselves into all kinds of anxious situations. Just give them a moment to play with an idea, and they're off on another anxiety trip.

But the good news is that you can also backtrack and rewind to a calmer place if you know how to apply *guided imagery*.

This technique worked for **Sylvia**. Tense thoughts fill Sylvia's every waking moment. From the time she springs out of bed in the morning to when the last gripping thought before restless sleep mercifully overtakes her, Sylvia thinks. She replays every anxious moment at work and dwells on each imagined mistake she's made during the day, turning them over and over in her mind. She visualises every flaw in her makeup, dress, and complexion. Images of incompetence, inadequacy, and unattractiveness flood her mind's eye.

To reduce the stress and anxiety that saturate the scenes in her mind, Sylvia decides to seek the services of a highly regarded counsellor. The counsellor teaches her several breathing techniques, but Sylvia still can't hold back the avalanche of anxious images. She tries progressive muscle relaxation, massage, and then music and aromatherapy, but all to no avail. Finally, the counsellor has an insight. 'Sylvia thinks in pictures. She needs *guided imagery!*'

Guided imagery harnesses your imagination to conjure up a pleasant, relaxing time or space. The best images incorporate all your senses. When visualising them, you see, hear, smell, feel, and possibly even taste. In Sylvia's case, her images were full of anxiety-arousing situations. When she tried other relaxation techniques, they failed, because anxious images still crowded unbidden into her mind. With guided imagery, however, the richness of the peaceful experience pushes aside all other concerns.

In this chapter, we show you how to heighten your imagination. Then we give you several scripts to experiment with in your mind. Feel free to rewrite them in any way you want. Finally, you can create your own special mental images.

Letting Your Imagination Roam

Some people, thinking of themselves as rather unimaginative, struggle to create pictures in their minds. These people generally feel uncomfortable with their drawing skills and have a hard time recalling the details of events that they've witnessed. Perhaps you're one of them. If so, using your imagination to relax and reduce your anxiety may not be the approach for you.

On the other hand, it just may be. Just remember that the vividness of the images does not predict the depth of relaxation that you can achieve. Guided imagery encompasses more than the visual sense; it includes smell, taste, touch, and sound. We can help you sharpen your ability to use all these senses.

We encourage you to give these exercises a go, but people all have different strengths and weaknesses, and you may find that one or more of these exercises just don't work for you. If you discover that guided imagery isn't for you, that's fine. This book discusses many other ways to relax.

To work with each of your senses, follow the three steps below before going through the guided imagery exercises in this chapter:

1. **Find a comfortable place to sit or lie down.**

2. **Make sure that you loosen any tight garments and shoes.**

3. **Close your eyes and take a few slow, deep breaths.**

Imagining touch

Imagery exercises work best if they incorporate more than one sense. Imagining bodily sensations enhances the overall experience of relaxing by using guided imagery. Try the following steps to see how this works:

1. **Imagine a huge, sunken bath.**

   What colour would you like it to be? How about the shape? Think about the lighting – candlelight, subtle spotlights, or would you prefer something else?

2. **Picture yourself turning on the tap and feeling the water coming out.**

   You can feel that the water is cold and wet as it pours over your hand. Gradually, the temperature increases to what is just perfect for you.

3. **The bath fills, and you can mentally see yourself pouring bath oil in and swirling it around.**

   You can feel how silky the water becomes.

4. **You imagine putting your foot in the water.**

   The water feels just a bit too hot at first, but you find that the warmth soothes you after you slowly lower your whole body into the bath.

5. **You lie back and luxuriate in the silky, smooth, warm water.**

   You can feel it envelop you as the warmth loosens all your muscles.

Were you able to feel the sensations: the wetness and the silky warmth? If not, don't despair. You can heighten the power of your imagination by spending just five minutes a day actively participating in a real experience and then concentrating on storing that experience in your memory. Try one or more of the following exercises each day for five days in a row. You can also experiment with other exercises. Just be sure to focus on touch.

- ✔ **Hold your hands under running water. Experiment with different temperatures.** Notice how your hands feel. Better yet, fill the basin and submerge your hands to conserve water.

- ✔ **Rub oil or moisturising cream on your hands and wrists.** Pay attention to all the feelings.

- ✔ **Take a warm bath and notice the sensations of wetness, warmth, and silkiness.** Focus on all your bodily sensations.

- ✔ **Soak a face-cloth in hot water, squeeze it out, and press it to your forehead.** Notice the warmth and the texture of the cloth.

- ✔ **Sit in front of a fire and notice where the heat hits your body.** Experience the warmth.

After carrying out one of the above exercises, a few minutes later, try to conjure up in your mind what the sensations felt like. The following day, do the exercise, wait five minutes, and then recall the sensations. Each day, gradually extend the length of time between the actual experience and recalling it.

Recalling sounds

You don't have to be a musician to appreciate music or to recreate it in your mind. Guided imagery often asks you to create the sounds of nature in your mind to enhance relaxation. Take the following steps to conjure up what an ocean beach sounds like:

1. **Imagine that you're lying on a beach.**

   You can hear the ocean waves rolling in one after the other. In and out. The soft roar soothes and relaxes. In and out.

2. **In your mind, you hear each wave rolling in. The sound rises to a crescendo and then the wave breaks gently onto the beach.**

   A brief moment of quiet follows as the next wave prepares to roll in. A few seagulls cry out as they fly overhead.

Were you able to hear the sea and the gulls? You can improve your ability to recreate sounds in your mind by actively experiencing the real thing beforehand. Try some of the following exercises for just five minutes a day for five days. You may also think of some other ways to practise listening to sounds with your mind's eye.

- ✔ **Listen to a short passage from a favourite song.** Play it several times and listen to each note. Tune in and really concentrate.

- ✔ **Sit in a chair in your lounge and just listen.** Disconnect the phone and switch off the music system and the television. Closing your eyes and listening carefully, notice every sound that you hear. Perhaps it's the traffic outside, a dog barking, the wind, or the house creaking.

- ✔ **Listen to the sound of yourself eating an apple, a celery stick, or a carrot.** Not only is it good for you to eat such foods, but you'll also hear interesting sounds. Eat slowly and hear each crunch. Notice the initial sharp sound of biting and the more muted chewing sounds.

As you did previously, wait a few minutes then try to hear the sounds in your mind. Hear them again. Don't worry if you can't do it. With practice, you're likely to improve. Each day, gradually increase the length you pause between the actual experience and recalling it.

Conjuring up smells

Dogs have a far better sense of smell than we do. They seem to know exactly which bush on their walk needs remarking. We're pretty sure that they know exactly which rival dog did what to which bush. Perhaps it's a good thing that our sense of smell isn't as good as theirs!

But smell has a powerful influence on people as well as dogs. Certain smells alert us to danger – such as the smell of smoke or burning food. Others, such as the aroma of your favourite baked delight or the perfumed scent of a loved one, conjure up pleasant memories and feelings. See whether this description brings a smell wafting into your mind:

1. **Imagine that you're walking across a field of newly mown grass.**

   It's late spring and the first time you've smelled cut grass this year.

2. **You can smell the sweet fragrance of the freshly cut grass.**

   The smell evokes memories of warm, carefree summer days.

3. **You stretch and breathe deeply.**

   A pleasant, refreshing feeling engulfs you.

How does this scene smell in your mind? Smell is often not as easy to consciously reproduce with your imagination as other senses. That may be because a description of smell is more difficult to put into words. However, with practice, you're likely to improve. Try a few of these activities to help you develop your imagination's sense of smell:

- ✔ **Make a cup of hot chocolate – the reduced calorie version if you prefer.** Before drinking it, spend a minute taking in the aroma. Focus on inhaling the smell as you take each sip.

- ✔ **Bake rolls or croissants.** Don't worry; you can buy the ready-made kind that you pop onto a baking tray. Sit in the kitchen while they bake. Open the oven door a couple of times to intensify the experience.

- ✔ **Visit a department store, go to the perfume counter, and test several different scents.** Try to describe the differences to yourself.

After a few minutes, try to remember what smell you experienced. Increase the gap between smelling and recalling the scent by a few minutes every day. Don't worry if you find this difficult; many people do.

Remembering tastes

Which foods do you associate with comfort and relaxation? Many people think of chicken soup or herbal tea. Do you pile the butter and jam on your toast when you're really stressed or occasionally indulge in ice cream – especially the one with chocolate and caramel swirls threaded through rich vanilla? Perhaps you're a chocoholic. Are you salivating yet? If not, try playing out this imaginary scene:

1. **Imagine an exquisite chocolate truffle.**

   You're not sure what's inside, but you look forward to finding out.

2. **In your mind, you take the truffle to your lips and slowly bite off a little piece.**

   The rich, sweet chocolate coats your tongue.

3. **You can imagine taking another bite and detect a creamy, fruity centre.**

   You never tasted anything so rich and delectable, yet not overpowering. The sweet but slightly tangy cherry flavour fills your body with satisfaction.

Could you taste the truffle in your imagination? Perhaps you found the taste easier to imagine than the smell. Either way, you can improve your ability to recall tastes with practice. Try one or both of these exercises:

- ✔ **Pick your favourite pastry – sweet or savoury, it's your choice.** You don't have to bake it from scratch; you can buy it ready-made if you prefer. First, explore and taste the pastry with the tip of your tongue. Take a little bite, and hold it in your mouth, then move it to different spots on your tongue. Start chewing slowly, and notice all the different flavours mixing together.

- ✔ **Open and heat up a tin of your favourite soup.** Pour a little into a cup or bowl. Put a small spoonful into your mouth. Make sure it's not too hot. Notice the variety of tastes on every part of your tongue.

You can do this taste-focusing activity with any food you choose. The key is to take some time and to focus. Savour the flavours and pay attention to the nuances – sweet, sour, bitter, or salty. Again, try to recall the tastes after about a minute. Then stretch the period between the actual experience and the recall to a little longer each time that you practise.

Painting pictures in your mind

Many of our clients report that scenes of anticipated disasters and doom enter unbidden into their imaginations. These scenes cause them more anxiety than actual disastrous events usually do. Visual imagery can fuel your anxiety or, alternatively, you can harness your visual imagination to help you quench the fires of anxiety. Try painting this picture in your mind:

Imagine you're at a mountain resort in late spring. The building's made of wood. Nestling into the hillside, it's surrounded by wonderful tall trees. Grey-blue smoke rises lazily from a chimney and curls away into nothingness.

Imagine you spent the day trekking through a forest. Now you're relaxing on the deck overlooking a valley lake ringed by mountain peaks.

The water in the lake is still; the dark blue surface reflects surprisingly clear images of the trees and mountains. The sun sinks behind a mountain peak, painting the clouds above in brilliant hues of red, orange, and pink. The mountains are still capped with winter snow. Dark green fir trees stand proudly on a carpet of pine cones and needles.

Mindfulness: Finding peace in the present

Our sense-sharpening exercises actually form part of a more powerful approach to overcoming anxiety called *mindfulness,* discussed in greater depth in Chapter 16. It's a technique that's been used for several thousands of years in both the secular and religious settings of the East. Mindfulness involves immersing yourself in the present with full awareness. When you fully attend to your immediate surroundings, catastrophic predictions about the future fade and anxiety diminishes. Mindfulness has only comparatively recently found its way into Western psychology. However, in the past few years, researchers have discovered that training in mindfulness can substantially enhance other approaches to anxiety reduction. We recommend that you work on sharpening your awareness of your experiences and then read Chapter 16 to discover more.

How did this scene look in your mind? If you practise sharpening your visual imagery, you'll become an expert eyewitness. Wherever you are, take a minute to inspect the view in front of you. It doesn't matter what it is. Scrutinise the image from every angle. Notice colours, textures, shapes, proportions, and positions. Then close your eyes. Try to recollect the images in your mind. Focus on every detail. You can practise this anywhere and at any time. It just takes a few minutes. Each day, delay your image retrieval a little longer after turning away from the scene that you just studied.

Full Sensory Imaging

The best and most effective guided imagery incorporates multiple senses – not necessarily every one, every time, but generally the more the better. If you aren't as adept at using certain senses, try to focus on employing your more-developed senses. We have a couple of imaginary scenes in the next section for you to try, which use most of your senses to recall an experience.

If you like our scenes, use them. Perhaps you'll want to make a tape recording of one or both of them. If you do, feel free to modify the scene in any way that helps you imagine it more vividly or feel more at peace. Record yourself reading the following sections and then play the tape back to help you relax. Perhaps you can play a recording of ocean sounds in the background as you read and record the 'Relaxing at the beach' exercise. Similarly, you can play a recording of forest sounds as you create your own recording of 'A forest fantasy'. Commercial recordings are also available.

Relaxing at the beach

1. **Imagine that you're walking barefoot along a sandy beach on a warm, sunny day.**

   The sand feels warm between your toes. Reaching the seashore, you paddle in the shallows and feel the cool, refreshing water lap over your feet. You smell the crisp, salty air and take a deep breath. Calmness settles over you.

2. **You walk a bit further and reach an area where rocks jut out into the surf.**

   A wave crashes onto the rocks and sends a fine mist high into the air; small droplets spray your face and feel delightfully refreshing.

3. **Seagulls glide effortlessly high above and then dive, skimming the surface of the water.**

   They look like acrobats of the sky, gracefully soaring in and out of sight. The surf and the seagulls orchestrate a soothing soundtrack. An old-fashioned wooden deckchair beckons to you further down the beach.

4. **You stroll over to the chair and stretch out on it.**

   The wood warmed by the sun is smooth and soothing against your skin.

5. **Magically, a frosted glass of your favourite drink appears beside you on a small side table.**

   Sipping and feeling the cold liquid fill your mouth and slide down your throat, you feel refreshed and satisfied, serene and content.

6. **You look towards the horizon, where a couple of sailing boats float lazily in the distance.**

   You feel the warm sun bathe your skin; at the same time, a gentle breeze cools your skin to a perfect balance. You've never felt so relaxed in your life.

7. **You lie back and close your eyes.**

   You can feel all the muscles in your body let go. You feel totally relaxed but alert at the same time. Nature's beauty fills you with awe, melting your worries away.

A forest fantasy

1. **Imagine that you're walking through pine trees and brush.**

   The sap of the trees gives off a sweet, pungent aroma. You hear the branches rustle in the breeze. Sunlight filters through the branches of the trees, making shadows that dance across the ground.

2. **Your feet feel the spring in the path – a path that is covered with years of fallen leaves.**

   You hear a stream burbling in the distance.

3. **You reach into your backpack, take out a container of cold water, and sip.**

   As you sip, you feel at peace and start to really relax. You hear birds overhead.

4. **As you climb, the trees begin to thin.**

   You reach a stream, its clear water flowing swiftly over and around the small rocks in its bed. You bend down to touch the water; it's cold, clean, and pure.

5. **You splash some ice-cold water over your face and feel cleansed.**

   Just ahead, you notice a grassy meadow, filled with wild flowers. The flowers' fragrance gently fills the air with sweetness.

6. **You reach a grassy, soft spot and sit down.**

   From here, you can see for miles into the distance. The air is pure and clean. The sun feels warm on your skin. The sky is a brilliant blue; a perfect backdrop to the few white, fluffy clouds.

7. **Sleepiness overtakes you and you lie down.**

   You can feel your entire body relaxing. Your everyday concerns seem trivial. All that matters is the moment. You cherish the experience of your connection to the earth.

Customising Your Own Images

You may want to create your own imaginary journey. It can be to somewhere that you've been before or somewhere you've never seen. You can be alone or have anyone you want there with you. Your companions will do whatever you want – it's your choice. Try a few different scenes to see how they work for you. Many people use guided imagery to help them go to sleep. Others use these images to help them relax before a stressful event, such as taking a test. We have a few helpful hints for designing your own guided imagery for relaxation:

- ✔ The most important thing is that you enjoy yourself.

- ✔ Be creative; let your mind go wild, coming up with any scene that may feel good to you.

- ✔ Use multiple senses – the more the merrier.

- ✔ Add descriptive details. Some people try and think of words as well as pictures. If you're one such person, consider using a thesaurus for rich adjectives.

Imagining a positive outcome

Athletes commonly use images to reduce their performance anxiety. In addition, many of them create images of success. For example, a gymnast may envision himself making a perfect dismount off the balance beam, over and over. Or a runner may see herself pushing through pain, stretching her legs out for a first-place finish, again and again. Various studies indicate that imagery can give an athlete an extra boost.

Imagery is great for children too. For example, children who suffer from recurring tummy pain often miss school and other activities. A study in 2006 used guided imagery and progressive muscle relaxation for this problem and found that the children said they had less pain and also that they missed out on fewer activities.

Another way to use imagery is to face your fears in a less stressful way than meeting them for the first time in real life. You do this by repeatedly imagining yourself conquering your fears. We tell you more about exactly how to imagine yourself conquering your fears in Chapter 8.

✔ Make enough happen in your scene so that it lasts a little while. It takes some time to let your body relax.

✔ You may like to play soothing music or sounds in the background as you make your recording describing the scene.

✔ Be sure to include relaxing suggestions, such as 'I'm feeling calmer', 'My worries are melting away', 'My body feels relaxed', or 'My limbs are loose and limp and floppy'.

✔ Realise that no rights or wrongs exist when designing an image. Don't judge your scene.

✔ If it doesn't work for you, don't force it. You can find many other ways to relax.

Chapter 14

Relieving Anxiety with Herbs and Dietary Supplements

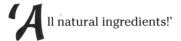ll natural ingredients!'

'Nature's way!'

Advertising slogans like these sound healthy and appealing, especially so to people who are unhappy about swallowing synthetic chemicals to reduce anxiety. People often think that supplements and herbs grown naturally in the wild can safely decrease anxiety without causing any distressing side effects. No wonder vitamin, herb, and other supplement sales have soared in recent years. In fact, a report in 2004 found that one in three people in the UK spends over £20 a month on herbal remedies – that's £126 million per year in total in the UK.

In this chapter, we tell you about herbs and supplements sold to reduce anxiety. But more importantly, we share the latest information about the effectiveness of these strategies, including warnings about their possible disadvantages and dangers.

Tell your doctor about any so-called natural products that you consume for any purpose whatsoever. Your GP needs to know this information in order to help you avoid unintentionally mixing medication into a potentially dangerous concoction. A qualified medical herbalist is also able to advise you.

Searching for Supplements

Dietary supplements include vitamins, amino acids, minerals, enzymes, metabolites, or botanicals that reputedly enhance your health and/or your body's functions. These supplements appear in many different forms, such as capsules, powders, tablets, teas, liquids, and granules. You can buy supplements over the Internet or from your local chemist, supermarket, or health food shop.

The claimed benefits of supplements include improved immune systems, enhanced sleep, stronger bones, more flexible joints, pain relief from arthritis, sleep improvements, greater sexual response, cancer cures, and overcoming anxiety.

People seek supplements often because they assume that they're safer than prescribed drugs. That's not necessarily true. Supplements are not considered to be drugs in the UK, and therefore are not subjected to the same level of scrutiny as most medication. Before a prescription drug can come to market, the manufacturer must conduct clinical studies to establish the safety, effectiveness, dosage, and any possible dangerous incompatibility with other medications. The UK Medicines and Healthcare Products Regulatory Agency (MHRA) doesn't require clinical trials to establish the safety of herbs. Instead, after a supplement makes it to market, the only way it will be removed is if enough consumers suffer serious side effects and complain to the right agencies, which can trigger an MHRA investigation and possible decision to withdraw the herb from sale.

Another serious problem with supplements is that untrained salespeople often make recommendations for their use. The advice of sales assistants varies widely in usefulness. Fortunately, healthcare professionals who are also interested and trained in the safe and effective use of supplements can help. Doreen's story isn't all that unusual.

A young salesperson, apparently bursting with health, smiles at **Doreen** as she enters the health food shop. Doreen tells him that she would like to find a natural remedy to help her calm down. She reports difficulty concentrating, poor sleep, and always feeling on edge. The young man nods and suggests a regime of vitamins and supplements to build up her resistance to stress, improve her concentration, and ease her symptoms of anxiety.

Pulling bottles off the shelves, he tells her, 'Some vitamin B complex to build you up; C to fight infections. Here are some amino acids – L-lysine and tyrosine – and a compound, 5-HTP. Minerals: calcium, zinc, potassium, and magnesium. Kelp nourishes, and you should make sure that you take vitamin B6 and niacin to improve your sleep. The herbs you may find useful are Californian poppy, limeflower, vervain, and wild lettuce. Oh yes, maybe some SAM-e to improve your mood. St John's wort can help with anxiety, stress, premenstrual syndrome, chronic fatigue, depression, and chronic pain, plus it's useful for helping you sleep and may overcome those winter blues. Other herbs are hops, passion flower, valerian, lemon balm, and chamomile. Now, take these at least an hour before you eat. Eat carbohydrates with these, not protein. And this one needs to be taken just before bed.'

The bill comes to £187, and Doreen goes home feeling a bit overwhelmed. One day at work, after ingesting a dozen pills, Doreen runs to the bathroom to vomit. A concerned friend asks her what's making her sick. Doreen tells her about all the supplements that she's taking. Her friend suggests that Doreen seek the advice of a qualified medical herbalist, homeopath, or naturopath; she explains that these professionals attend a four-year, full-time training programme and must pass a rigorous exam.

Doreen visits a naturopathic practitioner who advises her to dump the majority of her purchases in favour of a multiple vitamin and mineral supplement and one herb supplement. The practitioner also discusses several relaxation strategies, exercise routines, and self-help books. Within a few weeks, Doreen feels like a new person.

Drink and drugs: A potent brew

It's pay-day, and **Harry's** mates invite him down to the pub for a few beers. 'Sure,' he says. 'I can't stay too long, but I could do with a couple of beers; it's been a tough week.' Harry finishes off two halves of beers over the course of two or three hours. He stumbles a bit as he gets off the bar stool, and a friend asks whether he's okay. Harry reassures the friend that he's sober. After all, he only had two halves.

Driving home, Harry drifts into the wrong lane for a moment but swerves back into his lane. Just then, he hears a siren behind him. A few moments later, he sees police lights flashing. Puzzled, he pulls over. The police are sure Harry is drunk, but a breathalyser test registers his blood alcohol level as well below the legal limit. What's going on?

Harry recently complained to his GP that he was feeling stressed in his job. His doctor prescribed a low dose of anti-anxiety medication and warned Harry not to take too much and that it could be addictive if he wasn't careful. Harry found the medication useful, and it calmed him a bit, but the medication didn't quite do the trick. A friend recommended two herbs to try. Harry figured that would be a great, natural way to enhance the prescribed drug, and that herbs certainly couldn't hurt him. To add up Harry's intake, he had combined two anxiety-alleviating herbs, a prescription drug, and alcohol. He was lucky that the police pulled him over. Harry could have ended up in a serious accident, harming himself or others.

Don't forget, even moderate alcohol consumption, combined with anti-anxiety agents, can intensify sedative effects to the point of substantial impairment and even death. *Be careful!*

Viva vitamins and minerals!

Chronic stress taxes the body. The results of several studies link mood disorders to vitamin deficiencies, and especially severe deficiencies may make your anxiety worse. Therefore, many experts recommend a good multivitamin supplement.

Make sure that a supplement includes all the B-complex vitamins, particularly B1, B2, B6, and B12. In addition, experts recommend increasing your vitamin C and E intake. Low levels of the mineral selenium have been linked to anxiety and a depressed mood, so look for selenium in a multivitamin. Finally, calcium is often suggested for its reputed calming effect. Most experts believe that including magnesium with calcium is best because the minerals work *synergistically* so that together, the total effect is greater than that of each mineral on its own.

A review of a number of studies in 2006 looked at pre-menstrual syndrome and the effects that different substances – including calcium, magnesium, vitamin B6, evening primrose oil, *Vitex agnus castus, Ginkgo biloba,* and St John's Wort – had on it. The authors concluded that magnesium and evening primrose oil studies produced conflicting results, while there was substantial evidence that calcium and vitamin B6 are effective. They added that while there was not enough evidence to reach conclusions on the use of *Ginkgo biloba, Vitex agnus castus,* and St John's Wort, it did appear that these may be effective.

Can vitamins and minerals cure your anxiety? That's not likely. However, they may just help to keep your body in better shape for handling the stresses that come your way. Just take care and don't take huge quantities. Even vitamins can produce toxic effects at very large doses.

Sifting through the selection of supplements

If you search the Internet and your local health food shops, you can probably find over a hundred supplements advertised as antidotes for anxiety. But do they work? Only a few, it seems. The following have some evidence supporting their value as possible anxiety axes:

✔ **SAM-e:** Claimed to relieve the pain and stiffness of osteoarthritis and fibromyalgia, this amino acid occurs naturally in the body. It may also help treat depression and anxiety. However, research on this supplement remains scant. SAM-e appears to increase levels of serotonin and dopamine in the brain, which may theoretically alleviate anxiety.

Possible side effects, such as gastrointestinal upset, nervousness, insomnia, headache, and agitation may result, but again, little is known about the possible long-term effects.

Don't take SAM-e if you have bipolar disorder (manic depression) or severe depression. SAM-e may contribute to mania, which is a dangerous euphoric state that often includes poor judgement and risky behaviours.

✔ **5-HTP:** This popular supplement is a compound that increases the levels of serotonin in the brain. Serotonin plays a critical role in regulating mood and anxiety. Some evidence also exists that 5-HTP may increase the brain's natural pain-relievers, *endorphins*. (See Chapter 10 for more on endorphins.) Unfortunately, only limited research has been conducted on 5-HTP. These studies suggest that 5-HTP may reduce anxiety somewhat.

The most widely reported side effects of 5-HTP include nausea, drowsiness, and dry mouth. Other side effects are relatively rare, but these include headache, dizziness, and constipation.

Do not take 5-HTP if you are also taking another antidepressant. Also, avoid it if you have tumours or cardiovascular disease.

A number of practitioners of alternative medicine also frequently recommend the supplement gamma-aminobutyric acid (GABA). This supplement may have a mild tranquilising effect, but little data is available to substantiate that claim. In addition, some practitioners suggest that magnesium may improve circulation and muscular relaxation, and some evidence exists to back up this claim.

Hunting for Helpful Herbs

In the past decade or so, people have flocked to health-food shops, supermarkets, and chemists, and now the Internet in search of safe, natural remedies for their anxiety. Herbs promise to decrease symptoms of stress without potential side effects. Unfortunately, the vast majority of herbs today are sold by sincere, well-meaning sales staff who know little about their products, other than what's on the label or the manufacturer's flyers. But there are also several hundred herbalists in the UK with extensive training in the safe use of herbal therapy.

Herbs that have traditionally been used to calm the nervous system include valerian *(Valeriana officinalis)*, chamomile *(Matricaria recutita)*, passion flower *(Passiflora incarnate)*, limeflowers *(Tilia europea)*, lemon balm *(Melissa officinalis)*, vervain or verbena *(Verbena officinalis)*, pasque flower *(Anemone pulsatilla)*, scullcap *(Scutellaria lateriflora)*, and centaury *(Erythraea centaurium)*.

Valerian, St John's wort, and chamomile, among others, have experimental evidence behind them to show that they reduce anxiety-related symptoms. In the following sections, 'Valerian' and 'St John's wort', we tell you about important cautions, safety data or the lack thereof, and the latest findings concerning these herbs. Most of this research was conducted in Europe, where interest is particularly high, as opposed to the US.

Investigating Valerian

Valerian is a herb that is native to Europe and Asia. The word comes from the Latin term meaning 'wellbeing'. It has been traditionally used to promote sleep and relieve anxiety, nervous restlessness, and digestive problems. Like many herbs, valerian is used extensively in Europe, and is now gaining in popularity in the US.

Effectiveness

A number of studies with control groups that were given a placebo suggest that valerian enhances the quality of sleep for insomniacs. One study compared valerian with a prescription sleep aid (oxazepam) and found it equally effective.

A few controlled studies support valerian's use for the treatment of anxiety. A review in 2007 examined 36 patients with anxiety problems who were given valerian, diazepam, or a placebo. Results showed that according to the clinician's rating of the patient's anxiety, valerian and diazepam were equally effective, but no more or less effective than the placebo – something the patients took, which they thought had an effect, but had no active ingredients. Patients tolerated valerian and diazepam equally well. However, the review concluded that additional studies with larger numbers of patients are necessary before drawing conclusions about the effectiveness and safety of valerian as a treatment option for anxiety disorders.

Dosages

Specific recommended doses for the use of valerian for anxiety reduction aren't available as yet. However, for the treatment of insomnia, taking between 400 and 900 mg is generally recommended. The quality and purity of valerian products varies widely. Products with valerenic acid are considered to be somewhat superior.

It is safe to take valerian with other herbs, such as chamomile, lemon balm, and passion flower for sleep, and with St John's wort for anxiety. One excellent product available over the counter contains motherwort (*Leonorus cardiaca*), vervain, valerian, and passion flower.

Cautions!

Valerian appears to be a relatively safe herb. However, you shouldn't take valerian if you have liver problems or are pregnant or breastfeeding. Rare side effects can include stomach upset, headaches, and infrequently, liver damage. If you take too much, you may experience confusion, hypersensitivity, insomnia, or even hallucinations. Valerian may interact with other drugs at high dosages, so take care when combining valerian and medications.

Sizing up St John's wort

St John's wort *(Hypericum perforatum)* is a shrubby perennial with bright yellow flowers. Traditionally it was used by the ancient Greeks and Romans, who believed that St John's wort could deter evil spirits. The flowering tops of St John's wort are used today to prepare teas and tablets containing concentrated extracts. The herb has found new and widespread popularity as a natural antidepressant.

Effectiveness

St John's wort is most frequently used to treat mild depression. It has been used to treat other conditions associated with depression, including anxiety, stress, pre-menstrual syndrome, chronic pain, and seasonal affective disorder (SAD). It can help promote sound sleep.

Dosages

Choose preparations that contain 0.3 per cent hypericin. Like a prescription antidepressant, St John's wort needs to build up in your body's tissues before it becomes effective, so be sure to allow at least four weeks to determine whether it works for you. Take St John's wort with or after meals.

Cautions!

St John's wort is not to be used during pregnancy or breastfeeding or when being treated with therapeutic ultraviolet light. Hypericin can cause photosensitivity when ingested even in very small amounts, so people with fair skins are advised to avoid prolonged exposure to sunlight while taking St John's wort. Always consult your doctor before taking prescribed antidepressants and St John's wort together.

Waiting for the verdict on other herbal remedies

Many other herbal remedies for anxiety appear in books, magazines, and shops. Advertising promotes these as safe, effective methods. But beware;

many of these herbs haven't been subjected to scrutiny for effectiveness or safety. We suggest that you avoid these because so many other anxiety-reducing agents and strategies work without dangerous side effects.

Research on the use of herbs taken by pregnant or breast-feeding mothers has almost never been conducted. That's because no one wants to take any chances of harming the foetus or newborn baby. You should probably avoid all herbal products if you are pregnant or breast-feeding. At the very least, consult your doctor or a qualified medical herbalist before taking any herbs or supplements. We just don't have enough information to justify the risk.

On the other hand, we don't think you need to be overly alarmed about drinking a little herbal lemon balm or limeflower tea from time to time. Most of these teas contain relatively small amounts of the active ingredients and are unlikely to pose a threat. But if you really want to overcome your anxiety with herbs or supplements, use the ones with the most research backing their claims.

You may be curious about other herbs often recommended for anxiety reduction. Table 14-1 presents a quick overview of the most popular herbs.

Table 14-1	Herbs Which May Be Helpful	
Herb	*Research*	*Dangers*
Chamomile	Insufficient research to make reasonable conclusions about its effectiveness for anxiety reduction. This is one of the safest herbs.	Rare, severe allergic reactions possible if used topically (rubbed onto the skin). Should not be taken by those who have severe allergies to ragweed.
Ginkgo biloba	Research is insufficient to make reasonable conclusions about its effectiveness for anxiety reduction. Limited data suggests that it may improve short-term memory and/or your thinking ability. It may have limited usefulness for those with mild Alzheimer's or dementia.	Side effects can include stomach upsets, anxiety, insomnia, and bleeding complications. Do not take with other blood-thinning medications or before or after surgery.
Lemon balm	Widely used for the relief of anxiety and bodily tension. Research supporting its efficacy is scarce, but lemon balm has been used for centuries.	Appears to be relatively harmless.

Herb	Research	Dangers
Hops	Used for restlessness and insomnia. Insufficient research to support these assertions.	Don't use if you're depressed.
Ginseng	Often suggested for stress and fatigue. Although many consumers swear by it, research has generally failed to support its effectiveness. A few studies suggest it creates a sense of wellbeing.	Among chronic, heavy consumers, hypertension, excitation, and insomnia have been reported. It may interact with a variety of other drugs. Consult your physician or herbalist if you take any other medications.
St John's wort	Usually promoted for use with depression, but also recommended for alleviating anxiety. A number of studies on depression indicate it may have some value. Its use for anxiety isn't supported as yet, although most antidepressants decrease anxiety to some extent.	Don't take it if you're taking another anti-depressant medication, the contraceptive pill, immunosuppressive or chemotherapy drugs, or warfarin. Side effects include oversensitivity to sun, stomach upsets, restlessness, and headaches. May interact badly with wine or cheese.

People have used herbal remedies for thousands of years. Many remedies work extremely well. In fact, a significant number of prescription medications are derived from herbs. You may want to try out some of the herbs for your anxiety. We recommend that you read the literature about each herb carefully to make an informed choice before then purchasing herbs from a reputable dealer.

If you have severe anxiety, don't rely exclusively on herbs. You should consult a professional for therapy and/or medication. Inadequately treated anxiety is a serious problem.

Don't forget that herbs and supplements are not regulated in the same way that medicines are. For a medicine to be licensed it must be proven to be effective and safe in trials and then monitored in use for unknown side effects. These monitoring systems just do not exist in the same way for herbs and supplements. Often the evidence for the effectiveness of a herb is of poor quality and conflicts with other claims, so you can't know whether the herb or supplement does what the manufacturer says it does. In the world of herbal remedies, the systems that exist for medicines to ensure consistent strength, purity, and freedom from contamination do not exist.

Chapter 15

Prescribing Peacefulness

· ·

· ·

*T*he last several decades have witnessed an explosion in new knowledge about emotions, mental illness, and brain chemistry. Scientists recognise changes in the brain that accompany many psychological disorders. New and old drugs tackle these chemical changes, and using these drugs has both advantages and disadvantages.

This chapter helps you make an informed decision about whether to use medication for your anxiety. We give you information about the most widely prescribed drugs and some of their more common side effects. Only you, in consultation with your doctor, can determine the best way to help yourself.

Making Up Your Mind about Medications

Deciding whether to take medication to manage your anxiety brings up a number of issues to consider. This decision isn't one to take lightly. You should consult with your therapist, if you have one, as well as your doctor. Before you decide on medication, what have you done to alleviate your anxiety? Have you read this book and tried to follow the recommendations? Have you

✔ Overcome the obstacles to change? (See Chapter 3.)

✔ Tracked your worries over time? (See Chapter 4.)

✔ Challenged your anxious thoughts, assumptions, and words? (See Chapters 5, 6, and 7.)

✔ Confronted your fears head on? (See Chapter 8.)

✔ Simplified your life? (See Chapter 9.)

✔ Exercised? (See Chapter 10.)

✔ Tried improving your sleep? (See Chapter 11.)

✔ Tried using relaxation? (See Chapters 12 and 13.)

✔ Practised mindfulness? (See Chapter 16.)

 With a few important exceptions, which we review in this chapter, we recommend that you go through the preceding list before starting on medication. Why? First, some research suggests that certain medication may actually interfere with the long-term effectiveness of the most successful treatments for anxiety. That's especially true of the techniques designed to confront phobias and fears directly through exposure (see Chapter 8). Secondly, if you try the strategies in the list, you may very well discover that you don't need medication. Many of our recommended anxiety strategies can establish long-term changes and positively affect your entire life.

The disadvantages of medication

You need to reflect on both sides of any important decision. Medication has both pros and cons. The disadvantages include

✔ **Addiction:** Some prescribed drugs can lead to physical and/or psychological dependency. Coming off them can be difficult, even dangerous, if not done properly. However, contrary to what some people think, most prescribed drugs are not addictive.

✔ **Uncertain long-term effects:** We don't really have good information on possible long-term effects with some of the newest medications.

✔ **Conflict with personal beliefs:** Some people just feel strongly that they don't want to take medication. That's fine, but sometimes there are good reasons to reconsider this view.

✔ **Potential incompatibility with pregnancy and breast-feeding:** Only a few drugs are recommended for women who are pregnant or breast-feeding. With many drugs, the potential effects on the foetus or baby mean they are just too risky.

✔ **Side effects:** Most medication can have a variety of side effects, such as stomach upsets, headaches, dizziness, dry mouth, and sexual dysfunction. Working with your doctor, it may take some time to find the right medication that will alleviate your anxiety and not have overly unpleasant side effects.

The advantages of medication

Sometimes medication makes good sense. When you've tried the recommendations in this book, consulted a qualified therapist (see Chapter 22 for advice on finding a good therapist), and tried out what they suggest, but you still suffer from excessive anxiety, it may be time to chat to your doctor about medication. In weighing the pros and cons, we suggest that you take a good look at the benefits that medications can offer:

✔ When you are seriously depressed as well as anxious, medication can sometimes provide faster relief, especially when you occasionally feel suicidal. Depressed thinking may interfere with psychological therapy, and a combination of psychological work and medication in significant depression is thought to be more effective than either alone.

✔ When anxiety severely interferes with your life, medication can sometimes provide relief more effectively than other therapies or lifestyle changes. Examples of such interference are:

- **Panic attacks** that occur frequently and cause frequent 999 calls and visits to accident and emergency departments.

- **Anxiety** that feels so severe that you stop going to work or miss out on important life events.

- **Compulsions** and **obsessions** (see Chapter 2) that take control of your life and consume large chunks of time.

✔ If you experience a sudden, traumatic event and are totally overwhelmed and feel unable to think, a short course of the right medication may ease your situation. Examples of traumatic events include

- The sudden death of a loved one

- An unexpected accident

- Severe illness

- An unexpected financial disaster

- A natural disaster, such as a flood

- Being the victim of a serious crime

- Being the victim of terrorism

 In rare circumstances, the sudden death of a loved one may cause such severe anxiety that medical treatment is necessary. Generally the feelings of distress, shock, and disbelief are a normal part of adjusting to the person's death, and some treatments (benzodiazepines; a group of group of drugs are also known as tranquillisers and sedatives) may delay this adjustment.

Peter's story is a good example of how medication can help some people get through a difficult but temporary period in their lives.

Peter worked in central London. On 7 July 2005 he was walking from Russell Square underground station to his office when he saw the number 30 bus ahead of him ripped apart in a violent explosion. He was far enough away to escape without serious physical injury, but he witnessed the terror and horror.

Over the following week, Peter had severe trouble sleeping, and mainly as a result of tiredness, he was unable to function at work. In addition, he couldn't banish the horrific images from his mind and experienced flashbacks to the event. He felt jumpy and on edge and was irritable with his family. Where possible, he tried to avoid going past the place where he had seen the explosion. Peter went to his doctor because everything felt unreal. His doctor told him that he was suffering from an *adjustment reaction*. This is a psychological reaction to profound change in a person's life, which is characterised by anxiety and depression. Peter's doctor added that if the symptoms persisted for another three months, therapy would be a good idea. However, the doctor said that a prescription for a short course of sleeping tablets may improve his sleep and help him cope with work.

Peter left the surgery feeling hugely relieved that he wasn't losing his mind, which is what he had feared. He understood that getting over the problem couldn't be done by somehow magically pulling himself together. He followed the doctor's advice, and having learned from his reading on the subject how avoidance was making things worse, he dealt with his problems and regained his full health and quality of life.

Understanding Medication Options

Today, doctors have a wide range of medications for the treatment of anxiety disorders. New drugs and new applications for older drugs are consistently being developed and licensed. Don't expect our list to cover every possible medication for anxiety. In addition, our review can't and mustn't replace professional medical advice.

If you decide to ask your doctor about medication, don't forget to discuss the following important issues, should they apply to you. Communicating with your doctor about these considerations can help avert a potentially disastrous outcome. Be sure to tell your doctor if you

- ✔ Are pregnant or plan to become pregnant
- ✔ Are breast-feeding
- ✔ Drink alcohol

✔ Take any other prescribed drugs

✔ Take any over-the-counter medication

✔ Take herbs or supplements such as St John's wort

✔ Take contraceptive pills (some medication for anxiety reduces their effectiveness)

✔ Have had any bad reactions to medication in the past

✔ Have any allergies

✔ Have any physical conditions, such as high blood pressure, cardiac problems, liver disease, diabetes, kidney disease, or epilepsy

Most drugs prescribed for anxiety belong to one of the following categories, which we discuss later in this chapter. In addition, we include some miscellaneous medications that are not covered by these categories.

✔ Antidepressants

- Tricyclic

- Monoamine oxidase inhibitors (MOAIs)

- Selective serotonin reuptake inhibitors (SSRIs)

- Newer or atypical antidepressants

✔ Atypical antipsychotics

✔ Benzodiazepines (minor tranquillisers)

✔ Beta blockers

✔ Miscellaneous tranquillisers

✔ Mood stabilisers and miscellaneous

You may think that some of these categories sound a little strange. For example, antidepressants are used to treat depression, and beta blockers are prescribed for hypertension – so these don't intuitively sound like families of drugs for the treatment of anxiety. But we'll show you that they can have a helpful role to play in the treatment of certain types of anxiety.

Antidepressants

Antidepressant medication has been used to treat anxiety for many decades. That makes sense, because anxiety and depression often occur together. And both problems appear to have some similarity in terms of their biological underpinnings.

Monoamine oxidase inhibitors (MAOIs)

MAOIs are the oldest type of antidepressant medication. They inhibit a substance that oxidises critical neurotransmitters in the brain, so more of these neurotransmitters remain available to effectively regulate mood. MAOIs are used infrequently because they can have serious side effects. The most serious of these side effects occurs when those who take this medication eat food containing tyramine. This combination can trigger a *hypertensive crisis:* a sudden sharp rise in blood pressure that if severe can lead to a stroke or – rarely – even death.

Unfortunately, many foods and some drinks contain tyramine – especially if old, preserved, or off. So if you're taking MAOIs, your diet mustn't include

- Alcoholic or de-alcoholised (low alcohol) drinks
- Avocados
- Broad bean pods
- Cheese
- Salami
- Meat or yeast extract or fermented soya bean extract – for example, Bovril®, Oxo®, or Marmite®
- Pickled herrings
- Food that is suspected of being stale or of going off, especially meat, fish, poultry, offal, and game

However, MAOIs can be effective when other antidepressants haven't worked. If your doctor prescribes one, he probably has a good reason for doing so. Make sure that your read the instruction leaflet carefully, watch what you eat, and avoid the foods in the preceding list. MAO inhibitors include phenelzine (Nardil®), tranylcypromine (Parnate®) and isocarboxazid (Marplan®).

Tricyclic antidepressants

Tricyclic antidepressants have many different effects including increasing the effective levels of the neurotransmitters norepinephrine and serotonin in the nerve synapses. After you start taking them, they can take anywhere from 2 to 12 weeks to reach maximum effectiveness. Usually people notice an improvement by two weeks and often a slight improvement is apparent after a few days. Sometimes friends and family notice the improvement before the sufferer does.

Tricyclic medication can have a number of side effects, including dizziness, weight gain, dry mouth, blurred vision, constipation, and interference with sexual function, most often difficulty reaching orgasm. Some of these effects resolve over time, but they can persist even after several weeks.

Nearly 30 per cent of patients stop taking this type of medication because of side effects. Even so, many of the problems described above also occur in anxious or depressed patients who don't take medication. In fact, in clinical trials in which patients with depression or anxiety took placebo medication (sugar pills with no chemical effect on the body), nearly as many stopped taking the placebo due to bodily symptoms that they thought were side effects as stopped taking the real medication due to genuine side effects.

Many doctors prescribe medication for anxiety disorders starting with a low dosage and slowly increasing it. They prescribe a very low dose initially in order for your body to adjust to the medication with minimal side effects. They gradually increase the dosage in order to minimise negative reactions. It can take a while to reach an effective dose this way, but you'll probably find yourself able to tolerate the medication more easily.

Even with careful regulation of dosage, tricyclics have lost some of their popularity and for many conditions been overtaken by the newer selective serotonin reuptake inhibitors (SSRIs) (see the next section for more on these). SSRIs have fewer of these side effects. Common tricyclic medications include

- Amitriptyline (Triptafen®)
- Clomipramine (Anafranil®)
- Dosulepin/dothiepin (Prothiaden®)
- Doxepin (Sinequan®)
- Imipramine (Tofranil®)
- Nortriptyline (Motival®)

Selective serotonin reuptake inhibitors (SSRIs)

SSRIs only became available around 30 years after the development of MAOIs and tricylic antidepressants. Despite frustration with the side effects from the tricylics and MAO inhibitors, reasonable alternatives were unavailable for many years. The pharmaceutical industry has since developed a number of alternative drugs.

The first of the SSRIs to be developed and licensed was Prozac®, which was followed by several similar drugs. The SSRIs increase the levels of the neurotransmitter serotonin at the nerve synapses by inhibiting the reabsorption of serotonin into the nerve cells. At first the SSRIs were thought to have few side effects. However, it is now clear that they can cause problems such as nausea and difficulty reaching orgasm. Rare, but serious, side effects include bleeding into the gut and confusion, particularly in the elderly.

Saving your sex life?

Many medications for the treatment of anxiety and depression can interfere with arousal and the ability to achieve an orgasm. The worst offenders in this group of medications are the selective serotonin reuptake inhibitors (SSRIs). Many people taking these medications are so pleased with their reduced anxiety that they hesitate to complain to their doctor about a side effect on their sex lives. Occasionally, when anxiety has caused premature ejaculation, for some people the delay in achieving orgasm caused by the SSRIs is not a problem and is even a benefit! Others are upset by the side effect, but just too embarrassed to mention it. However, this side effect is extremely common, and your doctor has no doubt had many patients report it. So go ahead and talk with your doctor if you are having difficulty achieving orgasm, because there's no need for embarrassment. Certain medications have a lower tendency to cause this side effect than others, so your doctor may recommend an alternative. Don't forget that depression or anxiety themselves can spoil your sex life, and effectively treating these problems can make a big difference.

Like other antidepressants, SSRIs are an effective treatment for various anxiety disorders. See Chapter 2 for a description of anxiety disorders, and Table 15-1, later in this chapter, for a listing of the popular SSRIs. Doctors prescribe SSRIs for

- Agoraphobia
- Generalised anxiety disorder
- Obsessive-compulsive disorder
- Panic attacks and panic disorder
- Post-traumatic stress disorder
- Social phobias

Among the medication options, SSRIs are generally considered the first choice for post-traumatic stress disorder.

Table 15-1	Popular SSRIs	
Name	**Most Frequent Side Effects**	**Precautions**
Citalopram (Cipramil®)	Headache, tremor, sedation, abnormal dreams, nausea, sweating, dry mouth, and problems with ejaculation.	Do not take citalopram with another antidepressant or St John's wort, which can have a potentially fatal interaction.

Name	Most Frequent Side Effects	Precautions
Fluvoxamine (Faverin®)	Headache, drowsiness, dizziness, convulsions, nausea, hepatotoxicity, decreased libido, and sweating.	Fatal reactions have been reported when taken with MAO inhibitors. Do not take with other antidepressants or St John's wort. Smoking and drinking reduce its effectiveness.
Paroxetine (Seroxat®)	Headache, sedation, tremor, nausea, sweating, and decreased libido.	Fatal reactions have been reported when taken with MAO inhibitors. Do not take with other antidepressants or St John's wort. When taken with warfarin, can increase bleeding.
Fluoxetine (Prozac®)	Headache, nervousness, insomnia, tremor, nausea, diarrhoea, dry mouth, sweating, and decreased libido.	Do not take with other antidepressants or St John's wort. Can cause a paradoxical increase in obsessive-compulsive disorder when taken with buspirone.
Sertraline (Lustral®)	Headache, insomnia, agitation, male sexual dysfunction, diarrhoea, nausea, constipation, tremor, and fatigue.	Fatal reactions have been reported when taken with MAO inhibitors. Do not take with other antidepressants or St John's Wort.

Newer antidepressants

Newer types of antidepressants target other important neurotransmitters by themselves or in conjunction with serotonin. They are starting to look fairly promising for the treatment of various anxiety disorders.

As with most of the medications for anxiety, antidepressants should generally be avoided when pregnant or breast-feeding. Consult your doctor for the best alternatives.

Currently, some of the more widely prescribed designer antidepressants are listed in Table 15-2.

Table 15-2		Newer antidepressants	
Name	*Uses*	*Most Frequent Side Effects*	*Precautions*
Venlafaxine (Effexor®)	Recently approved for the treatment of generalised anxiety disorder (GAD), but likely to be useful in treating other anxiety disorders, including panic disorder and post-traumatic stress disorder.	Sweating, insomnia, weakness, dizziness,dry mouth, sexual dysfunction, abnormal vision, migraine, swelling, raised blood pressure, and weight loss or gain.	Those with hypertension should generally avoid this medication, and special care should be taken when prescribed for children and/or the elderly. Those with bipolar disorder (manic depression) run the risk of triggering a euphoric, manic phase. This drug can increase the effects of alcohol, opioids, sedatives, and antihistamines.
Mirtazapine® (Zispin®)	This medication has shown some effectiveness with panic disorder, generalised anxiety disorder (GAD), obsessive-compulsive disorder, and post-traumatic stress disorder (OCD). It is sometimes used when SSRIs haven't worked.	They include weakness, dizziness, drowsiness, diarrhoea, dry mouth, increased appetite, urinary retention, blurred vision, abnormal dreams, and weight gain.	Those who've had hypersensitivity to tricyclic antidepressants and those with convulsive disorders or in recovery from a myocardial infarction shouldn't use mirtazepine. It can increase the effects of alcohol, barbiturates, and benzodiazepines. Fatal reactions have been reported when taken with certain antihistamines. Reports also indicate the possibility of hypertensive crisis when this drug is taken with MAOIs.

Benzodiazepines

Better known as *tranquillisers* or *anxiolytic* (anxiety reducing) drugs, the benzodiazepines were first introduced over 40 years ago. At first, they seemed like the perfect medication for a host of anxiety problems. Unlike the antidepressants,

they work rapidly, often banishing symptoms within 15 to 20 minutes. Not only that, they can also just be taken on an as-needed basis when having to deal with an especially anxiety-arousing situation, such as confronting a phobia, giving a speech, or going to a job interview. The side effects tend to be less disturbing than those associated with antidepressants.

For around 20 years after their introduction, they were seen as safer than barbiturates, with a lower risk of overdose. They rapidly became the standard treatment for most of the anxiety disorders. They appear to work by enhancing the actions of a natural brain chemical, GABA (gamma-aminobutyric acid) that inhibits the excitability of nerve cells. About 40 per cent of the millions of neurons throughout the brain respond to GABA, so this means that GABA has a general quietening influence on the brain: It is in some ways the body's natural hypnotic and tranquilliser. What could be better?

Well, it turns out that the benzodiazepines do have a major problem: addiction. Nothing's perfect after all. Even though they are very effective, *tolerance* to the drug often develops. This means that you require increasingly higher dosages to achieve the same effect. *Dependency* (physical and psychological) also develops, meaning that you need to take the drug just to feel normal. Without the drug, you feel worse than you did before starting it. Memory problems are another possible side effect.

As with many addictions, the withdrawal from benzodiazepines can be difficult and even dangerous. Furthermore, if you have had anxiety for a long time, you can take benzodiazepines, but when you stop taking them, your anxiety is almost bound to return. Experiencing a rebound anxiety upon withdrawal that's more severe than that experienced before taking the drug is possible, and this is more likely if you have taken benzodiazepines for a long time.

Older people increase their risk of falls if they take benzodiazepines. And falls among the elderly too often result in hip fractures. In addition, a recent report suggested that benzodiazepines may double the risk of becoming involved in a road traffic accident. That risk rapidly escalates when benzodiazepines are taken in combination with alcohol. In fact, benzodiazepines are particularly problematic for those who have a history of substance abuse. These people readily become addicted to these medications and are at greater risk of combining alcohol with their medication.

It initially seemed logical to prescribe benzodiazepines for those who had suffered a recent trauma. Indeed, these medications have the potential to improve sleep and reduce both arousal and anxiety. However, a study published in the *Journal of Clinical Psychopharmacology* (1998) found that the early and prolonged administration of benzodiazepines after a trauma actually appeared to increase the rate of full-blown post-traumatic stress disorder later. (See Chapter 2 for more information about post-traumatic stress disorder.) They may also interfere with your ability to adjust following a bereavement.

It also seems logical that combining benzodiazepines with some of the various changes in behaviour or thinking that can reduce anxiety (see Chapters 5, 6, 7, and 8) would make for a useful, synergistic combination that could yield better outcomes than with either approach by itself. Yet some studies have found that the risk of relapse is increased when these medications are combined with changes in thinking and behaviour. In the long run, it appears that for most people, learning coping strategies to deal with their anxiety seems better than seeking pharmacological solutions, especially with respect to the benzodiazepines.

Nevertheless, the benzodiazepines have been popular in the treatment of anxiety disorders. In part, that may be due to the rapid relief from anxiety and low side-effect profile of the drugs. These medications sometimes have an important role to play, especially for *acute* (short-term) stress and anxiety, as well as for those for whom other prescribed drugs haven't helped. However, a greater awareness of the potential for causing dependence exists and the development of tolerance, and consequently most doctors are reluctant to use benzodiazepines for long-standing conditions.

We urge caution with the use of benzodiazepines. Table 15-3 lists the more commonly used members of the family.

Table 15-3	The Benzodiazepines (Tranquillisers)	
Trade Name	**Most Frequent Side Effects**	**Precautions**
Lorazepam (Ativan®)	Dizziness, drowsiness, confusion, blurred vision, and unsteadiness.	Avoid if you have a history of drug abuse or narrow-angle glaucoma. Can increase the effects of alcohol and other central nervous system depressants.
Chlordiazepoxide (Librium®)	Drowsiness, confusion, blurred vision, dizziness, loss of co-ordination, and nausea.	Avoid with history of drug abuse (but often used to facilitate alcohol withdrawal) or narrow-angle glaucoma. Can increase the effects of alcohol and other central nervous system depressants.
Oxazepam	Same as for diazepam.	Same as for diazepam.
Diazepam (Valium®)	Dizziness, drowsiness, blurred vision, fatigue, and confusion.	Same as for chlordiazepoxide.
Alprazolam (Xanax®)	Dizziness, drowsiness, confusion, headache, tremors, blurred vision, and unsteadiness.	Same as for lorazepam.

Miscellaneous tranquillisers

A few miscellaneous tranquillisers are chemically unrelated to the benzo-diazepines and thus appear to work rather differently.

You should know that in addition to these miscellaneous tranquillisers, other types of tranquillisers are available. Furthermore, new types of anti-anxiety drugs are under development, and some are undergoing clinical trials. Some of these are fast acting, and it is hoped that they may have fewer of the unde-sirable side effects that have been found with the benzodiazepines.

For the time being, Table 15-4 lists two anti-anxiety medications that your doctor may prescribe.

Table 15-4	Miscellaneous Tranquillisers		
Name	*Uses*	*Side effects*	*Precautions*
Buspirone (Buspar®)	Buspirone belongs to a class of chemical compounds referred to as *azaspirones*. It has been studied the most for the treatment of generalised anxiety disorder, but may have value for treating various other anxiety-related problems, such as social phobia and post-traumatic stress disorder.	Usually mild and include, headache, drowsiness, dizziness, and nausea.	Shouldn't be taken in conjunction with MAOIs as it may raise blood pressure. Combining with alcohol is best avoided. Before operating a motor vehicle, be certain that the medication doesn't have an adverse affect on performance, judgement, and co-ordination. Care should be taken for those who have impaired liver or kidney function.
Hydroxyzine	An antihistamine which has the side effect of sedation. In addition to its use as an anti-histamine for allergic reactions, such as hives and itching, it has also been used to treat various kinds of anxiety and tension-related problems in the past, although this is less common now. It's fast-acting and takes effect within 30 minutes.	Dizziness, drowsiness, dry mouth, and confusion.	May increase the effects of alcohol and other central nervous system depressants. Take great care when driving or operating machinery. Not considered appropriate for long-term use and special care needed when prescribed for the elderly.

Beta blockers

Because anxiety can increase *hypertension* (high blood pressure), perhaps it's not surprising that a few medications for the treatment of hypertension also reduce anxiety. Chief among these are the so-called beta blockers that block the effects of noradrenaline (also known as norepinephrine) and adrenalin (also known as epinephrine).

Noradrenaline and adrenalin are released by a part of the nervous system called the *sympathetic nervous system.* The sympathetic nervous system is important in controlling some body functions such as blood pressure and heart rate, and beta blockers can help lower blood pressure. The sympathetic nervous system is also important in preparing the body to respond quickly to danger, the so called *flight or fight* response. In the flight or fight response your heart beats faster, you hyperventilate, your muscles become tense and ready for action, your pupils become wide to see more clearly, your hair stands on end, and lots more besides! You can see that many of the features of the flight or fight response are similar to symptoms of anxiety and panic attacks. Refer to Chapter 2 for more on the flight or fight response.

Thus beta blockers, which block many of the effects of the sympathetic nervous system, can help reduce many of the physical symptoms of anxiety, such as shaking, trembling, rapid heartbeat, and blushing. In the treatment of anxiety, their usefulness is primarily limited to specific phobias such as social anxiety and performance anxiety. See Chapter 2 for more on specific phobias. Beta blockers are popular among professional musicians who often use them to reduce their performance anxiety prior to an important concert or audition. Two beta blockers, propanolol hydrochloride (Inderal®) and atenolol (Tenormin®), are most frequently prescribed for these purposes. See Table 15-5 for more information.

Table 15-5	**Beta Blockers**		
Name	*Uses*	*Most Common Side Effects*	*Precautions*
Propranolol	Short-term alleviation of stage fright, public speaking nerves, test anxiety, and social anxiety. Often given as a single dose prior to a performance.	Usually rare. However, drowsiness, light-headedness, lethargy, insomnia, nightmares, fatigue, mental changes, nausea, and problems with erections may occur. More seriously, may aggravate asthma or make blood pressure drop excessively.	People who suffer from asthma, chronic lung disease, diabetes, certain heart diseases, myasthenia gravis, and those with very low blood pressure shouldn't take this drug.

Name	Uses	Most Common Side Effects	Precautions
Atenolol	Similar to propranolol, but the effects last longer. Atenolol is also often given as a single dose prior to a performance.	Same as propranolol, but less frequent.	Same as propranolol.

Atypical antipsychotics

As the name 'antipsychotic medication' suggests, this type of medication is used to treat psychosis. A psychotic illness is one in which the sufferer may have hallucinations, delusions (false beliefs, held with absolute conviction), or very jumbled thinking. However, over the years, antipsychotic medications have proved very helpful in treating severe anxiety.

In recent years, a new class of antipsychotic medication has become available, called *atypical antipsychotic medication*. The older typical antipsychotic medications all worked mainly on the dopamine system in the brain. The new atypical antipsychotics act on a wider range of neurotransmitter systems, usually a combination of serotonin and dopamine. They also have a much lower risk of certain side effects and they can be used to treat a far broader range of problems than just the psychoses. The atypical antipsychotics are sometimes given in combination with selective serotonin reuptake inhibitors (SSRIs). When used to treat anxiety-related problems, these medications are usually prescribed at far lower doses than when used for psychotic disorders.

The primary use of atypical antipsychotics to date has been for the treatment of severe cases of post-traumatic stress disorder and also for obsessive-compulsive disorder (see Chapter 2). Evidence to date suggests that these drugs can improve outcomes for people who haven't done well on other medications for these problems. Studies haven't been conducted on the use of these medications for other anxiety disorders, such as generalised anxiety disorder, agoraphobia, and panic disorder (see Chapter 2). However, case reports are mounting that suggest they may be beneficial for these problems as well. Soon, controlled studies may back those reports up with stronger evidence.

Who can prescribe medication?

Only medically qualified doctors – such as GPs and psychiatrists – can prescribe the medication discussed in this chapter. Some specialist nurses can also prescribe certain medications. Other professions are gradually being allowed to prescribe specific medications, with appropriate further training, and in the future clinical psychologists may also have limited prescribing rights.

Here's the low-down on how those who prescribed are trained for the job:

✔ Psychiatrists and GPs first go through medical school to qualify as doctors, which takes at least five years. This is followed by a two-year foundation programme working in hospitals and general practice. For GPs, this is followed by a further three years specialising in general practice, or for psychiatrists by six years specialising in psychiatry.

✔ Clinical psychologists usually graduate from university with a first class degree and then complete a minimum of three years on a postgraduate doctoral clinical psychology degree. They undertake training in the science of human behaviour and the treatment and diagnosis of emotional and mental disorders.

In the UK, GPs prescribe the majority of psychotropic medications and treat most patients with psychiatric problems. With more severe or complicated problems, they will refer to psychiatrists. Psychiatrists have a detailed knowledge of psychotropic medications and should probably be consulted if medication issues are complicated. Clinical psychologists and other trained psychological therapists generally provide psychological therapy.

So with the potential of these particular drugs, you may think that they would quickly become the treatment of choice for most anxiety disorders. Well, just hold your horses. It's not likely to happen in the near future because these drugs occasionally have some especially distressing side effects. Possibly the most disturbing are the *extrapyramidal symptoms* (EPS), which can include a wide range of problems, such as

✔ Abnormal, uncontrollable irregular muscle movements in the face, mouth, and sometimes other body parts

✔ An intense feeling of restlessness

✔ Muscle stiffness

✔ Prolonged spasms or muscle contractions

✔ Shuffling gait

The good news is that these EPS appear to occur much less often with the newer atypical antipsychotic medications as opposed to the older, traditional antipsychotic medications. However, other side effects that you should know about are weight gain and reduced sex drive, and some antipsychotic medications can cause an increased in the hormone prolactin. In women, increased prolactin can interfere with periods and cause small amounts of milk production, while in men it may cause breast enlargement. Because the risk of EPS is relatively low, those with severe anxiety disorders for whom changes in behaviour or thinking (see Chapters 5, 6, 7, and 8), or other medications haven't helped sufficiently, may want to consider using these new anti-anxiety medications.

However, given the risks, those with relatively milder anxiety problems would probably want to avoid these atypical antipsychotic medications. We discuss three of the new antipsychotic medications in Table 15-6. Others are under development.

As with most of the medications for anxiety, these should generally be avoided when pregnant or breast-feeding. Consult your doctor for the best alternatives.

Table 15-6	Atypical Antipsychotics		
Name	*Uses*	*Side Effects*	*Precautions*
Risperidone (Risperdal®)	Treatment of severe post-traumatic stress disorder and obsessive-compulsive disorder. May effectively treat other severe anxiety disorders as well. Reduces symptoms of anxiety, depression, and anger when added to selective serotonin reuptake inhibitors (SSRI) medications.	The most common ones include drowsiness, dizziness, weight gain, nausea, and constipation. However, it can also lead to extrapyramidal symptoms, such as muscle stiffness, involuntary movements, shuffling gait, and breast swelling.	Those with seizure disorders should avoid this medication. When starting risperidone, you may get dizzy if you stand up too quickly or have hot baths because the drug may cause your blood pressure to drop. Various serious drug interactions can occur with over-the-counter medications. The drug may increase the sedative effects of alcohol and other central nervous system depressants.

(continued)

Table 15-6 *(continued)*

Name	Uses	Side Effects	Precautions
Olanzapine (Zyprexa®)	Little demonstrated its effectiveness for anxiety disorders, but may be effective for the treatment of severe post-traumatic stress disorder and the anxiety experienced among Alzheimer's patients. Effectiveness with other anxiety disorders is promising but remains to be demonstrated with controlled trials.	Probably one of the most easily tolerated antipsychotic medications, but does cause dry mouth, constipation, weight gain, and drowsiness.	Avoid alcohol or other central nervous system depressants. May interact with various over-the-counter medications.
Quetiapine (Seroquel®)	Little research supports this medication as a treatment for anxiety problems, but the drug may have significant potential.	Dizziness, dry mouth, headache, back pain, weight gain, nausea, constipation, and headache. The drug may have the lowest risk of extrapyramidal side effects of all atypical antipsychotics.	Those with liver disease or seizure disorders should take special care with this drug.

Mood stabilisers

These medications are usually prescribed for the treatment of bipolar disorder (sometimes called manic depression) or epileptic seizures. However, when standard treatments haven't worked, doctors sometimes find mood stabilisers useful for their patients' anxiety. Specific drugs in this category include valproate (Epilim®) or valproate semisodium (Depakote®) and carbamazepine (Tegretol®).

Chapter 16

Practising Mindful Acceptance

*H*as your car ever been stuck on a muddy road? What happens if you put your foot down hard on the accelerator when the wheels start to spin? They spin even faster, the mud flies everywhere, and the rut gets deeper. Anxiety can be like that: The harder that you try to break free, the tighter it seems to grip.

But then you have a flash of insight. You let the car rock back into the rut, and you gently accelerate at the right moment. If the wheels start to spin again, you gently ease off on the pedal, letting the car rock back. Eventually, you find a rhythm that gets you out of the rut and onto more solid ground – until you get stuck in the next rut, that is! But at least you get somewhere, a little at a time, and you do it by *accepting* the idea of going backwards for a while.

In this chapter, we explain how to use *acceptance* as one way to get out of your anxiety trap. Threads of what we call *mindful acceptance* appear throughout this book. We weave the threads together to form a tapestry. We show you that acceptance helps you to stop spinning your wheels, so that you can calmly consider productive alternatives. We discuss how too much concern with ego and self-image can make seeing the way out difficult. We also explain how living in the present provides a route to a more balanced life.

About Turn! Accepting Anxiety?

So how come, after showing you how to get rid of your anxiety, we tell you to mindfully accept it? Isn't this book supposed to be about *overcoming* anxiety?

Well yes, of course we want you to overcome your anxiety. But the paradox of anxiety is that the more you feel you must rid yourself of it, the more anxious you feel. The more that your anxiety disturbs you, the more it will ensnare you.

Have you ever seen a dog with a choke chain being taken for a walk on a lead? The harder the dog pulls, the tighter the collar squeezes. There seems no way out, so the dog pulls even harder at first. Eventually, the dog realises that the only way to deal with the situation is to stop fighting against it.

Anxiety mimics the squeezing of a choke chain. The more that you struggle, the more trapped you feel. Insisting that your anxiety go away this second is a guaranteed way to increase it!

Taking a dispassionate view

Anthropologists study the behaviour and culture of human beings. They make their observations objectively from a dispassionate, scientific perspective. We want you to view your anxiety like an anthropologist would, and be coolly detached.

Wait for the next time that you feel anxious. Study your anxiety and all that goes with it and prepare a report that conveys what anxiety feels like in your body, how it affects your thoughts, and what it does to your actions. Don't judge the anxiety, just observe it. Then, being as objective as possible, answer the following questions:

- Where in my body do I feel tension? In my shoulders, back, jaw, hands, or neck? (Study it and describe how the tension feels.)
- Are my hands sweating?
- Is my heart racing? If so, how fast?
- Do I feel tightness in my chest or throat?
- Do I feel dizzy? (Study the dizziness and describe it.)
- What am I thinking? Am I . . .
    - Making negative predictions about the future?
    - Making a mountain out of a molehill?
    - Turning an unpleasant event into a catastrophe?
    - Upset about something that's outside my control?
- What is my anxiety telling me to do?
    - To avoid doing something that I want to do?
    - That I need to be perfect?
    - That I have to cover up my anxiety?

Martin's story provides a good example of how your powers of observation may help you come to grips with your anxious feelings.

Martin, a 38-year-old NHS manager, experienced his first panic attack three years ago. Over the next three years, his attacks increased in frequency and intensity, and he even started to miss work on days when he feared having to chair staff meetings.

Martin is now working with a therapist to decrease his panic. The therapist notices that Martin's perfectionism means he demands instant improvement. He reads everything the therapist recommends and tries to do every task perfectly. The therapist, realising that Martin needs to slow down, gives him a new homework task: to pretend to be an anthropologist on a mission to study his anxiety. Here's the report Martin wrote:

> I started noticing a little shortness of breath. I thought, 'Here it comes again!' Then my heart began to race. I noticed it was fast but not quite as fast as when I exercise. I wondered how long it would last. Then I noticed that my hands were sweating. I felt a little nauseous. I didn't want to go to work. I could almost hear the anxiety telling me that I'd feel much better if I stayed home because if I went to work, I'd have to talk to a room full of angry consultants. I know I have to tell them about the new duty rota system. They're not going to like it. They'll probably tear me to pieces. What an interesting image. I've never really been torn to pieces, but my image is amazing! If I get too anxious, I bet I'll start talking nonsense, and I'll look like a complete idiot. This is interesting too. I'm making incredibly negative predictions about the future. It's funny, as I say that, I feel just a tiny bit less anxious.

Martin discovered that letting go and merely observing his anxiety helped him deal with it. Rather than attack his anxious feelings and thoughts, he watched and pondered his experience by really trying to reproduce the sense of scientific curiosity that anthropologists seem to have.

Just give me a break!

Tune into your mind's internal chatter. If you're like most people with anxiety, your chatter too often consists of a stream of self-criticism. Here are some examples of the internal critic at work:

- ✔ I'll never get it done on time.
- ✔ I'll look like a fool.
- ✔ I can't stay in control.
- ✔ I'll make a total mess of everything.
- ✔ I'll be sick.

> ✔ What if I become hysterical and run out of the room screaming?
>
> ✔ I hate myself.
>
> ✔ I'm a lousy parent.
>
> ✔ Nobody will like me.
>
> ✔ I'm stupid.
>
> ✔ Any minute now, they'll all find out what a fake I am.
>
> ✔ If people really knew me, they wouldn't like me.

Now, look at those statements and try changing the word *I* or *me* to *you* and change *I'll* to *you'll*. Say them out loud as though you're talking to someone you know well, perhaps a friend. Can you really imagine telling a friend

> ✔ You'll look like a fool.
>
> ✔ You're a lousy parent.
>
> ✔ Nobody will like you.
>
> ✔ I hate you.

It's doubtful. The odds are that you'd never say anything like this to a friend or, for that matter, to a mere acquaintance, and yet that's what many people say to themselves time and time again.

It's as though a judge is sitting in your mind, but this judge has no mercy and no compassion. This judge evaluates every flaw or shortcoming and ignores genuine mitigating circumstances.

Listen to your mind chattering away. When you hear the judge, try replacing the comments with a more compassionate, self-forgiving approach. Be a friend to yourself.

Tolerating uncertainty

Anxious people usually loathe uncertainty. If only they could control everything around them, they wouldn't worry as much. That's probably true; if you could control everything, you wouldn't have much to worry about, would you?

The rather obvious flaw in this approach lies in the fact that life consists of constant uncertainty and a degree of chaos. In fact, a fundamental law of physics states that, even in so-called hard sciences, absolute certainty is nonexistent. Accidents and unforeseen events happen.

For example, you don't know the day and time that your car will break down. You can't predict the stock market, although many try. Bad things happen to good people all the time. Even if you spent every moment of your waking life trying to prevent illness, financial difficulties, and loss of loved ones, you couldn't do it.

Not only is the task of preventing future catastrophes impossible, you can easily ruin most of the present time if you try. Think about it. If you thoroughly check your car's engine before every journey, if you scrimp and save every possible penny for retirement, if you never eat ice cream because of the fat content, if you overprotect your children because you worry that they'll get into trouble, if you wash your hands every time that you touch a door knob, if you never take a single little risk, then what would your life be like? Probably not much fun.

And worry doesn't change what will happen. Some people think that if they worry enough, bad things won't occur. Then, because bad things don't happen to them on most of those worry days, they feel as if their worrying has paid off. But just think about it. Has worry, by itself, ever actually prevented anything from happening in the history of humanity? Not once.

Find out how to embrace uncertainty. It can make life both interesting and exciting. When you find yourself feeling anxious, ask yourself whether this is about attempting to control the unpredictable.

Some people try to play the stock market. They may try to increase the interest on their savings or attempt to build up a pension. They constantly worry about their investments, watching their stocks and shares on a daily basis. They scan the newspaper for financial information that may possibly help them know when to buy and sell at just the right moment.

Now, we're certainly not trying to give you financial advice. Others far more knowledgeable than us can do that for you. However, we do know that most studies indicate that precise attempts to predict the stock market are doomed to fail. By all means invest in the stock market, if you can afford to take a small risk. But fretting and worrying about your investments on a daily basis is likely to harm your health and probably won't increase your wealth.

Let go of your need to predict and control. Of course, take reasonable precautions about your health, family, finances, and wellbeing, but when worry about the future erodes the present enjoyment of your life, it has gone too far. Appreciate uncertainty and live well today.

Making patience a virtue

When you think about patience, what comes to mind? Calmness, acceptance, and tolerance. When you become anxious, try to be patient and kind with yourself and say to yourself:

- ✔ Okay, I'm feeling anxious. That's just the way I'm feeling.

- ✔ Like other feelings, anxiety comes and goes.

- ✔ Let me experience my anxiety.

In the story of Janine that follows, Janine's contrasting reactions, first with impatience and then with patience, provide an example of how you too can turn your impatience into patience.

Janine begins to feel anxious on the way to work in the morning. She leaves home at 8 a.m. and usually gets to work on time at 9 a.m. On most days she's even about five minutes early, but occasionally she gets stuck in a traffic jam and is a few minutes late. This seems to be one of those days.

- ✔ **The impatient Janine:** Traffic is at a standstill, and increasing anxiety churns acidly in Janine's stomach. Sweating, gripping the steering wheel, she begins lane-hopping to try to cut through the traffic a bit faster. Drivers hoot in irritation. She hates starting her day like this. She can't stand the anxiety and tries to banish it, but she fails. She visualises her boss commenting on her late arrival, and her colleagues all looking at her. Anxiety turns to anger as she beats herself up for not leaving earlier.

- ✔ **The patient Janine:** Traffic is at a standstill, and anxiety churns in her stomach. Clutching the steering wheel, she fights the urge to change lanes. She notices and accepts the anxiety in her body, thinking, 'I may be late, but I'm normally on time or early. My boss and colleagues know that. I can feel my anxiety, but it's okay to experience it. How interesting. And if I arrive a few minutes late this morning, that's still all right.'

In the second scenario, the anxiety dissipates because Janine allowed herself to feel it without judgement or intolerance. She connected to her present situation with patience.

Like everything else, making patience a habit takes practice. You build your tolerance for patience over time. Like building muscles by lifting weights, you can build the patience muscles in your mind a little at a time.

Reaching serenity or at least getting closer

Accepting anxiety involves a variety of related attitudes – being non-judgemental, tolerating uncertainty, letting go of the need for absolute control, and patience. Realise that acceptance isn't the same as resignation or total surrender.

> Acceptance simply means appreciating that you, just like everyone else, have strengths and limitations. You realise that you'll never completely get rid of your anxiety. Rather, over time, you figure out how to deal with it and give up being anxious about feeling anxious. Only then will it stop overwhelming and dominating your life.

Letting Go of Ego

Everyone wants to have a positive self-image. Bookshops and libraries display hundreds of books about how to develop and improve the way you see yourself. You may think that having a positive self-image would decrease your anxiety, and the more positive the image, the less anxiety you would experience. It seems logical at first sight.

However, self-image doesn't always work that way. In fact, an over-inflated *ego,* or view of yourself, can actually increase your anxiety, and may cause other problems too. Most positive human characteristics and qualities can turn into negatives when they reach extreme levels. For example, courage, generosity, conscientiousness, and trust all are wonderful traits. But too much courage can make a person reckless, excessive generosity can make you an easy target for the unscrupulous, excessive focus on work can leave insufficient room for pleasure, and excessive trust can mean you get taken for a ride. Perhaps our analogy of the inflated ego being like a balloon may help you understand the unexpected danger of too great an investment in ego or self-image.

Inflating and deflating the ego, or self-image, balloon

We think of self-image as being like a balloon. If it's too low then, like an empty balloon, it has no air; it's flat, deflated, and can't float. A deflated balloon isn't especially fun or useful. If your self-image is quite low, you probably spend time judging yourself harshly and negatively. Your energy probably suffers, and you may feel quite anxious about your perceived deficiencies.

An over-inflated ego or an exaggerated self-image, however, is like a balloon that's tightly stretched and so full of air that it's about to go pop. One tiny scrape and the balloon bursts. People with an oversized ego worry constantly about those scrapes. Any threat to their self-image causes considerable anxiety and sometimes anger. You can't do much in life without running into at least some threat to your ego. If your self-image balloon is too full of itself, those threats can appear especially ominous.

On the other hand, a balloon with just the right amount of air doesn't burst easily. It can bounce around joyfully and playfully. The balloon with the right amount of air doesn't worry much about bumping or bursting.

In a sense, both the deflated balloon and the one close to the bursting point are very concerned with their own state – their condition, worth, and vulnerability. The key to having just the right amount of ego or air in the balloon is to have *less* concern with yourself (along with more concern for others) and less worry about how you stand as compared with others, while still being aware of, and valuing, your positive qualities. When you can accept both your positive and negative qualities without being overly concerned about either, you'll have the right amount of air in your ego balloon. That isn't always so easy to do. It takes a solid focus on learning, striving, and working hard, though not working to excess.

It's not easy being a beginner

All too often, anxious people feel they must be perfect in order for others to like and accept them. No wonder they feel anxious. Nobody's perfect, and no-one ever will be.

Imagine a perfect woman. **Catherine** is perhaps as close to perfect as you can get. She always wears exactly the right outfit, her choice of colour is superb, and all her accessories match. She takes an evening class in interior design, and her home is absolutely stunning. She works out at the gym four times a week and eats only healthy foods. Her makeup is always immaculate. She invariably knows just what to say, never stumbles over a single word, and certainly never swears. She's kind to animals and has an almost infuriatingly positive outlook.

Would you like to go out for a drink or a coffee with Catherine? Does she seem like someone you'd like to invite to your spur-of-the-moment barbecue one summer weekend? Would you feel comfortable with her? Most people would probably feel intimidated at the thought of having her as one of their best friends.

Now think about one of your good friends with whom you like to spend time. Choose someone you particularly like and value, who you've known for a while. Picture that person in your mind and recall some of the good times you've spent together. Enjoy those images. Think about how much you appreciate this person and how your life has been enriched by the relationship.

Realise that you've always known about your friend's negative qualities and imperfections, yet you've continued to appreciate your friend. Perhaps you even find some of the flaws amusing or interesting. Maybe they give your friend colour. Thinking about the flaws isn't likely to change your opinion or feelings either.

Try applying the same principles to yourself. Appreciate your idiosyncrasies. They make you interesting and unique.

Be a friend to yourself. Notice your good and bad points. Find a way to accept yourself and see yourself as good enough, just the way you are.

Colin tried an exercise that helped him to see that shortcomings don't mean that people will disown you and walk away. Colin filled in the Appreciating Imperfect Friends exercise in Table 16-1, thinking about his friend Jack. In each column, he wrote about Jack's qualities and imperfections.

Table 16-1	Appreciating Imperfect Friends	
Positive Qualities	*Negative Qualities*	*Imperfections*
Jack is one of the funniest guys I know.	Sometimes Jack talks too much.	Jack's a little overweight.
He's always there for me.	Even though he's intelligent, sometimes Jack makes stupid decisions, especially about money.	Sometimes Jack drinks a bit too much.
Jack will help me any time I need it, no matter what.		He doesn't always listen to me.
I like the fact that Jack's really bright.		Jack has terrible taste in clothes.

Colin accepts Jack, warts and all. There's no-one else that Colin would rather spend time with, and Jack's the first person he would turn to in a crisis. Can Colin accept himself like he does Jack? That's much harder.

Try doing the exercise that Colin did. Think of a good friend you've known a while and write down what you like and enjoy about the person. Then list what about that person may be off-putting. Finally, write down the person's shortcomings.

If your friend filled out the same form about you, no doubt it would include some wonderful qualities plus some less-than-wonderful traits. But would your friend suddenly end the friendship because of your imperfections? Of course not; nobody is perfect. If we all disowned our imperfect friends, we'd end up with no friends at all.

Have you ever been done for speeding or had a parking ticket? It's so easy to beat yourself about it. 'Why did I do it? What an idiot! Now there's the fine – plus points on my licence – what a total twit I am!' Yet if it happened to your partner or friend, would your response be something along the lines of 'It can happen to anybody.'? It really is so important to treat yourself with the same compassion you show to others.

Self-acceptance is difficult. It's even harder to drop defensive barriers in response to criticism from others. Work out how to listen to criticism. Consider the fact that it may at least have an element of truth. Appreciate that portion of truth. If your partner says that you don't listen, perhaps that's true, at least some of the time!

Try acknowledging any elements of truth that the criticism contains. It may be true *sometimes.* Maybe it's partially applicable. Instead of putting up barriers to communication and problem solving, if you admit your faults, you're likely to actually strengthen relationships.

Sometimes criticism can be abusive. If the tone is hostile or aggressive, you don't need to put up with it. If someone is constantly criticising you, discuss it with a trusted friend. It may that the behaviour is totally out of order and unacceptable. You may be the victim of verbal abuse, and that's a different matter entirely.

Focusing on the Present Moment

In some ways, language represents the pinnacle of evolutionary development. Language sets humans apart from the rest of the animal kingdom. It's linked to all the arts and allows us to express complex ideas, plus it gives us the tools for creating solutions to problems. At the same time, the things we say to ourselves – the language we use – can cause us great distress. How come?

Like humans, dogs also get distressed. But for dogs, this usually only happens when they directly experience pain or discomfort. For example, dogs rarely enjoy going to the vet. More than a few dog owners have had to drag their dogs into the vet's surgery, pulling on the leash with all their might.

However, humans do what dogs would never do. Humans wake up dreading the events of the day that lies ahead. Dogs don't wake up at 3 a.m. and think, 'Oh no! Today's the day that I have to go to the vet! What's he going to do to me this time?'

And dogs have few regrets. Of course, they sometimes look pretty guilty when caught chewing on their owner's shoe. But one kind word and a pat on the head, and they've forgotten all about it. Some anxious people still remember the thank you note that they forgot to write to Aunty Betty six years ago.

Generally speaking, dogs seem much happier than us humans. Unless dogs have been horribly abused, they're usually happy and contented and sleep a lot. By contrast, humans worry a lot. They get anxious about a catastrophic future and dwell on their past transgressions.

When you bring possible future catastrophes as well as past regrets into the present, you're essentially using language to disconnect yourself from real-life experience. Doing so can totally spoil the enjoyment of your *present moments,* which make up the very time that you actually *live* your entire life! Consider the following example of Tony, who dreaded the amount of work that he believed he had to finish within the next five days:

Tony is a barrister. An important trial is coming up in five days. The thought of the amount of work he has to get through almost paralyses him. He also agonises over the possibility that his performance will lack brilliance. But most of all, he worries about getting to grips with the huge number of papers, briefs, depositions, and petitions that are involved in the trial. He knows that he'll be working from dawn to dusk with barely enough time to breathe.

The funny thing about it, though, is that after the trial is over, Tony realises that most of those five days turned out to be fairly enjoyable. He worried over the possibility of not completing his tasks, yet this had nothing to do with any of the actual work that he did. Most of the time that he was working, he actually felt pretty good. Not a single, individual moment felt *horrible* by itself.

The next time that you go over and over future or past events, tasks, or outcomes, try doing the following:

- ✔ Stay focused on each successive moment as you experience it.

- ✔ Spend a few minutes noticing all the sensations in your body at any given moment – touch, taste, smell, sight, and sound.

- ✔ When thoughts about the tasks ahead enter your mind, simply acknowledge the presence of those thoughts and try to move your attention back to the present.

- ✔ If thoughts about past failures or regrets enter your mind, notice the presence of those thoughts and move your attention back to the present.

- ✔ Remind yourself that *thoughts* about the past or future are only *thoughts,* they are not the reality.

✔ When you notice disturbing thoughts about the future or the past, try just observing them. Notice how interesting it is that your mind comes up with thoughts like these and then return to the present moment.

✔ Remember: Few present moments truly feel unbearable. It's simply our ability to ruin the present with thoughts about the future or past that disturbs us.

✔ Consider re-reading Chapter 5 about how distorted your thoughts can be, and work on making them more realistic. Then return to the present again.

In Chapter 5, we explained how to carefully analyse the way that anxiety can cause you to make negative, distorted predictions. Then we showed you ways of making more accurate predictions. Nevertheless, that approach can only take you so far. No matter how hard you work at it, you're likely to find negative thoughts popping into your head every now and then. When they do in spite of your best efforts to reframe them with more accurate predictions, go back to the last exercise. It can help you tune out the negative chatter.

We have another idea to help you stop paying attention to that stream of worries about future events:

1. Think about how many times you've made negative predictions in the past about some forthcoming event.

2. Then ask yourself how often those predictions came true. If you're not sure, keep a record of your negative predictions and see what percentage actually happen.

3. Of those forecasts that do come true, how often is it as bad as you anticipated? If you're not sure how often, keep a log for a while.

Most people tell us that at least 90 per cent of what they worry about never happens. Of the 10 per cent that does occur, less than one predicted event in ten is bad as they'd anticipated. That's far too much worry and way too many ruined present moments just to anticipate the few unpleasant occurrences.

Taking these predictions seriously is rather like listening to the weatherman on the television who tells you that blizzards, severe cold, and ice storms are forecast for each day. So you dutifully put on your heavy coat, gloves, and boots. Just one problem nags you, however. You know that 90 per cent of the time (in the scenario of negative predictions) the forecast is absolutely wrong, and the weather is sunny and warm. When the Met Office gets it almost right, the conditions are still seldom as bad as described. So you have spent all that unnecessary time overheating yourself into a state of discomfort, with no benefit. Perhaps it's time to stop listening to the weather report in your head. You can't turn the station off, but you can at least take the reports less seriously!

Making contact with the present

At this very moment, consider coming into direct contact with your experience. This is something many people have rarely done. Have no expectations about what this exercise is *supposed* to do. Just study what happens.

1. Notice how this book feels in your hands. Feel the smooth cover and the edges of the pages.

2. Notice how your body feels as you sit, stand, or lie. Pay attention to the way your skin feels when it makes contact with the surface below it.

3. Feel the muscles in your legs, your back, and your hands and arms as you hold the book.

4. Notice your breathing. Feel the air go in and out of your nostrils.

5. Notice any smells, whether pleasant or unpleasant. Think about how you may write a report about these smells.

6. If thoughts interrupt you, notice them. Don't judge them. Then return to noticing all your present sensations.

7. Hear any sounds around you. If you hear loud, obnoxious sounds, try *not* to judge them. Instead of thinking about how jarring they sound, study the nuances in the sounds. Imagine how you would describe these sounds to a friend.

8. If judgements enter your mind, observe how your mind just automatically comes up with these. Make no judgements about these thoughts or yourself.

9. Go back to focusing on the entire spread of present-moment sensations.

Now notice how you feel at the end of this exercise. Did you experience the sensations fully? What happened to your anxiety? Many people report that they feel little, if any, anxiety during this experience. Others say that their anxiety escalates.

If your anxiety increases during your first few attempts to connect with present-moment experience, don't worry. It happens for various reasons. Increased anxiety doesn't mean that you're doing something wrong. More than likely:

- You may have had little experience connecting to the present. Therefore, it feels strange.

- Anxious thoughts may interrupt you frequently. If so, more practice may help to reduce their impact and frequency.

- You may be under such overwhelming stress at the moment that putting this strategy into effect is unrealistic. If so, you may want to try other strategies in the book first.

Whatever you do, we recommend trying frequently to connect with present-moment experience.

Most anxiety and distress come from thoughts about the future or the past, not what's happening at this moment.

Mindfully noticing and enjoying life

As well as reducing anxiety, mindful acceptance can improve the quality of your life. When you're anxious, so much of your mental energy focuses on negative sensations, thoughts, and images that you miss much of life's simple pleasures.

Mindful eating

How many times have you eaten a meal and barely tasted it? Of course, if it tastes like cardboard, perhaps that's a good thing. However, most of the foods that we eat taste pretty good. It's such a pity to miss out on the full experience.

Choose a time to practise mindful eating. Be sure that you have longer than a ten-minute lunch break – though you won't have to spend all afternoon over it. Worrying thoughts may sometimes distract you. That's fine and normal. However, try merely noticing them. Rather than judge those thoughts or yourself, return your focus back to your eating, as shown in the following exercise:

1. Slow down and focus before taking a bite.

2. Look at your food.

3. Notice how it's displayed on your plate or bowl.

4. Observe the food's colours, textures, and shapes.

5. Take time to smell the aroma.

6. Put a small portion on your fork or spoon.

7. Before you take a bite, hold the food briefly under your nose and really notice the aroma.

8. Briefly put the food on your lips and then on the tip of your tongue.

9. Put the food in your mouth, but don't bite down for a moment or two.

10. Start chewing very slowly.

11. Notice how the taste and texture change with each bite.

12. Notice how the food tastes on different parts of your tongue.

13. Swallow the mouthful and notice how it feels sliding down your throat.

14. Follow this procedure throughout your meal.

15. Stay seated at the table with your meal for at least 20 minutes. If you finish eating before the 20 minutes is up, continue sitting until the full time is up, all the while noticing your surroundings and the sensations in your body.

Consider making mindful eating a regular part of your life. You'll feel calmer, enjoy your food more, and possibly even lose a little weight. Many weight-loss programmes suggest slowing your eating down. However, this approach does more. It enables you to fully experience your food. When your mind totally focuses on the present pleasure of eating, anxiety fades away.

Mindful walking

Look around at people walking to their various destinations. So often they rush frenziedly about like hamsters on an exercise wheel, not even aware of their surroundings. Rushing people, unlike hamsters, don't enjoy the exercise. Their minds fill with anxious anticipation and worries.

We have an alternative for you to consider. Mindful walking. You've probably tried taking a walk sometime when you felt especially stressed. It probably helped. However, mindful walking can help you even more. This is how it's done:

1. Pause before you start.

2. Notice the feeling of air going in and out of your nose and lungs. Breathe quietly for five breaths.

3. Begin walking slowly.

4. Notice the sensations in your leg muscles, your ankles, calves, and thighs. Spend a minute or two focusing only on these muscles and how they feel.

5. If troubling thoughts intrude, simply notice them. Watch them like clouds floating overhead. Don't judge them. When you can, refocus on your muscles.

6. Now, feel the bottom of your feet as they touch the ground. Try to notice how the heel hits first, then the foot rolls, and then you push off with the ball of your foot and toes. Concentrate on the bottom of your feet for a minute or two.

7. Bring yourself back to the present if troubling thoughts intrude.

8. Now focus on the rhythm of your walking. Feel the pace of your legs and the swing of your arms. Stay with the rhythm for a minute or two and enjoy it.

9. Feel the air flowing into your nose and lungs. Then breathe out and in again, taking notice of the rhythm of your breathing. Focus on nothing else for a minute or two.

10. Now pay attention to your feet, to your muscles, to the rhythm of your walking, and to your breathing. Shift your attention from one to the other.

11. Practise mindful walking for five minutes a day. Try it for five successive days. Then consider whether you want to make it a regular part of your life.

Enthusiasts extol the virtues of mindful walking. They claim it helps them reduce stress and become more serene. You can experiment with mindful walking in various ways. For example, try focusing on sights and sounds or focus on the smells as you encounter them. Play with this strategy and develop your own approach. There's no right or wrong way to being mindful.

Making Mindfulness a Part of Your Life

Some people read about mindfulness and worry about the time it can consume. They say that it sounds like living life in slow motion and complain that nothing can ever get done if they try living that way. As much as we think that living a little slower isn't a bad idea for many people, mindful acceptance doesn't require significant chunks of time.

Mindfulness entails a shift in thinking that decreases the focus on ego, pride, and control, while emphasising accepting the present with all its gifts and challenges. Being mindful acknowledges that uncertainty is inherent in life.

Making mindful acceptance a habit doesn't happen overnight. With practice, it can slowly permeate your life. Accept that you won't always stay in the present. Don't judge your attempts to live mindfully. When you see yourself living in the guilt-ridden past or anxious future, gently remind yourself to come back to the present.

Part V
Helping Others with Anxiety

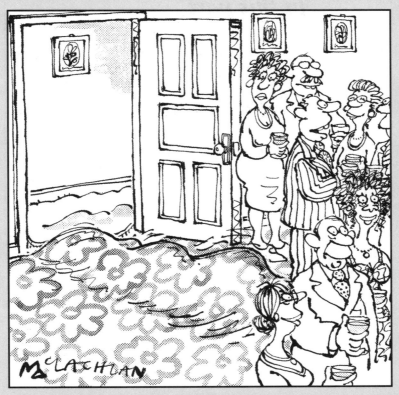

'Marjorie's decided to come to your party after all despite her social phobia.'

In this part . . .

We reveal that today's kids appear more anxious than ever before. Kids are anxious about both real and imagined fears. We help you distinguish between normal and abnormal childhood fears. Then you discover how to prevent your children from developing abnormal fears and what you need to do if they already have too much anxiety.

The final chapter in this part details what you can do when someone you care about has anxiety and worry. First, we help you find out if your loved one suffers from anxiety, and then we show you how to talk about it. Finally, we provide strategies for working together on the problem.

Chapter 17

Helping Your Children Fight Anxiety

*C*hildhood anxiety has grown to epidemic proportions during the past 40 to 50 years. Numerous studies confirm this alarming development, but one in particular is a shocker. Psychologist Jean Twenge compared symptoms of anxiety in today's children with symptoms in seriously disturbed children receiving hospital treatment in 1957. She reported in the *Journal of Personality and Social Psychology* (December 2000) that boys and girls today report a greater number of anxiety symptoms than psychiatric inpatient children reported in 1957.

Should these findings cause alarm? We think so. The statistics are disturbing enough in their own right, but when you consider the fact that anxiety disorders often precede the development of depression later in life, it raises concerns that the consequences of childhood anxiety may worsen in the years to come.

In this chapter, you discover the difference between normal and problematic anxiety in children. We explain that some childhood fears are completely normal, while others require intervention. In some cases, that intervention means getting professional help. Whether you need a professional or not, we show you a number of options you can try with your children to help them deal more effectively with their anxieties. Doing so may prevent more serious, long-term problems.

Separating Normal from Abnormal

So what's going on? Why do our children experience emotional turmoil? Of course, we all know the complexities and tensions of the world today – parents working longer hours, rapidly developing technologies, violence on television and in video games, and even terrorism. We also suspect that certain styles of parenting are partially responsible for the development of some difficulties. We discuss this in the 'Parenting precautions' section later in this chapter.

For the moment, what you as a parent need to know is how to distinguish the normal anxieties of childhood from abnormal suffering. Realise that the vast majority of children feel anxious at various times to one degree or another. After all, one of the primary tasks of childhood is to figure out how to overcome as many as possible of the fears that life creates for everyone. Successful resolution of those fears usually results in good emotional adjustment. You just need to know whether your children's fears represent normal development or a more problematic frame of mind that requires help. Look at Table 17-1 to get an idea of the anxiety that you can expect your children to experience at one time or another during their youth.

Table 17-1	Does Your Child Have an Anxiety Problem?	
Anxiety Problem	*When Anxiety is Normal*	*When Anxiety Should Go Away*
Fear of separation from mother, father, or carer	Common at ages 6–24 months. Don't worry!	If this continues with no improvement after 4 years of age, then you have some cause for concern.
Fear of unfamiliar adults	Common at ages 6–10 months.	Don't be too concerned unless you see this after 2–3 years of age. And don't worry about a little shyness after that.
Fear of unfamiliar peers	Common at ages 2–30 months.	If this continues without showing signs of reducing after 3 years of age, you have some cause for concern.
Fear or animals, darkness, and imaginary creatures	Common at ages 2–6 years.	If these fears don't start to decline by 6 years of age, you have cause for concern. Many children want a night-light for a while and that's fine; don't worry unless the fears are excessive.

Anxiety Problem	When Anxiety is Normal	When Anxiety Should Go Away
Fear of school	Mild to moderate school or childcare phobia is common at ages 3–6 years; it can briefly reappear when moving from infant to junior school.	This should decline and cause no more than minimal problems after age 6 years. A brief re-emergence during secondary school is quite common, but it should soon pass. If it doesn't, that may be a concern.
Fear of being judged by others	This fear almost defines adolescence. Most teenagers worry quite a bit about what others think of them.	It should gradually reduce as adolescence unfolds.

Table 17-1 gives you some general guidelines about common or 'normal' childhood fears. However, independent of a child's age, if fears seem especially serious and/or interfere with your child's life or schoolwork in a major way, they may be more serious and warrant attention. In addition, other anxiety problems in the 'Identifying the Most Common Childhood Anxiety Disorders' section later in this chapter – such as obsessive-compulsive disorder, panic attacks, or generalised, excessive worrying about a wide variety of fears – are not particularly *normal* at any age.

Tommy's troubles

Julie doesn't know what to do about her 7-year-old son, **Tommy.** Every day, she battles with him about going to school. At first, she thinks he really is ill, so she takes him to the GP. After a complete physical examination, the doctor reassures her that Tommy is healthy. The doctor encourages Julie to send Tommy to school and warns that if she doesn't, Tommy's behaviour is likely to worsen. He also adds that legal implications exist if children regularly miss school – parents can even be sent to prison!

'My tummy's sore,' whines Tommy. 'I don't want to go to school.'

'Now darling, you've missed so many days,' soothes Julie, 'you really should go today; you're not that sick.'

'But my tummy really hurts; it really, really does, Mummy.' Tommy begins to sob.

'You will go to school today,' Julie says firmly, grabbing Tommy by the hand. Tommy plants his feet and pulls away, screaming. Julie can't believe what he's doing. He actually seems terrified; Julie's never seen him behave this way before. Frantically, Tommy runs to his bedroom and hides in his wardrobe. Julie finds him huddled there, sobbing.

Tommy suffers from school phobia, a common but serious childhood anxiety disorder. Sensibly, Julie decides to seek further professional help.

If you have any doubts about the seriousness of your children's anxiety, you should consider getting professional advice. An educational or child psychologist or your family doctor should be well equipped to handle your questions, quite possibly in a single visit. Anxiety problems sometimes precede other emotional difficulties, so you should see someone sooner rather than later.

Identifying the Most Common Childhood Anxiety Disorders

Some fear and anxiety is normal for children. You can probably remember being afraid of the dark, monsters, or ghosts. However, other types of anxiety, while not always rare, do indicate a problem that you should address. We briefly review the more common types of problematic anxiety in children in the following sections. Then we tell you about the primary risk factors linked to these anxieties and, most importantly, what you can do about them.

Leaving parents: Separation anxiety disorder

As we showed in Table 17-1 in the preceding section, children frequently worry about separations from their parents when they're as young as 6 months to perhaps as old as 4 years of age. However, if children continue to be very frightened of separating after about the age of 4 years, they may need help, especially if the issues below apply to the child:

- Becoming very upset when thinking about or being separated from parents or carers

- Exaggerated worry about harm coming to parents or carers

- Refusal to go to school or participate in activities due to worries about separation

- Insisting on having a parent or carer accompany them to bed and stay until they fall asleep

- Frequent nightmares about separation

- Frequent physical complaints, such as headaches, stomach aches, and so on, when separated or separating from parents or carers

Among the various anxiety disorders, separation anxiety disorder is relatively common in children, but that doesn't mean it's normal. The average age it seems to start is around 7 to 8 years of age. The good news is that a large percentage of those with separation anxiety disorder no longer fulfil the diagnostic criteria for the disorder three or four years later.

The bad news is that quite a few children who have suffered from separation anxiety go on to develop other problems, especially depression. It's for that reason that we suggest prompt action if separation anxiety lasts longer than a couple of months and interferes with normal life.

Worrying all the time: Generalised anxiety disorder

Based on what we know today, generalised anxiety disorder (GAD) is probably fairly common among children and more common among older children than younger ones. It most often occurs around puberty and is characterised by

- Excessive anxiety and worry about school or family problems
- Physical symptoms, such as stomach aches, headaches, or loss of appetite
- Difficulty concentrating and/or irritability

Focusing on phobias: Specific phobias

Most young children at one time or another are afraid of the dark or monsters under the bed. So don't worry if your child has these fears unless the fear becomes so intense that it disrupts daily living in a significant way. The typical age that a *clinical* phobia (one which is severe and interferes with life, rather than earlier, minor fears) arises is about age 8 or 9.

Getting back to school

Children can develop anxieties and be reluctant to go to school. This can happen for many reasons. These include fear of separation from their parents or carers, which is very common when first starting school and even when changing schools. Other reasons include bullying and learning difficulties. In some children, anxiety can express itself though long-term incontinence.

If your child is reluctant or refuses to go to school, it's useful to arrange an appointment with the headteacher to discuss how to work together to overcome the problem. The first step is to identify the nature of the problem. In the case of soiling or wetting, your family doctor should be consulted, because this may be due to anxiety or to a physical problem. If necessary, the headteacher will refer the child and/or family for further specialist help, which may include an educational psychologist, child and families team, or a speech therapist. The headteacher will support the child and family throughout the process until the problem is overcome.

Specific phobias are exaggerated, intense fears that cause a child to avoid a particular object or situation. See Chapter 2 if you want more information on this type of anxiety.

Mixing with others: Social phobia

Some children are very shy. They seem to have been born that way, and relatives often make comments such as, 'He's just like his dad was at that age.' Sometimes, shyness decreases with age, but when shyness increases and causes a child to fearfully avoid social encounters in everyday life, your child may have a problem.

Social phobia usually doesn't get diagnosed until around 10 years of age. Signs generally appear at a younger age, but parents often have trouble distinguishing social phobia from shyness until then. You can pick up the signs sooner if you observe your children carefully. If their fears of unfamiliar peers or adults show no improvement whatsoever by age 3 or so, you may want to check with a professional as to whether the problem is serious. See Chapter 2 for more information about social phobia.

Anxious repetition: Obsessive-compulsive disorder

This type of anxiety is somewhat less common than separation anxiety disorder, GAD, specific phobias, and social phobias. Nevertheless, almost 1 in 50 teenagers has obsessive-compulsive disorder (OCD). Often beginning in childhood, OCD develops on average at around age 10. However, it can occur as early as 4 or 5 years of age.

Post-traumatic stress disorder among children

Post-traumatic stress disorder (PTSD) is thankfully rather rare in children. The symptoms are slightly different between children and adults. Like adults, children can get PTSD from abuse or other directly experienced trauma. (PTSD among New Yorkers increased after the September 11 terrorist attacks, and 9- to 11-year-olds were particularly affected). Also, like adults, children can develop PTSD from witnessing trauma happening to others, such as seeing a parent attacked.

Children with PTSD become restless, agitated, irritable, and have difficulty concentrating. Instead of nightmares and intrusive thoughts, children may act out their terror during play. They may have bad dreams, but these usually don't have content specifically relevant to the trauma. Like adults, they become anxious and alert to any possible sign of danger. They also tend to over-react to trivial incidents, such as being bumped into or criticised.

Obsessions are recurring, unwanted thoughts that your child can't stop. See Chapter 2 for more details. Some of the most common obsessions among children include

- ✔ Excessive fear of intruders
- ✔ Fear of germs
- ✔ Fear of illness
- ✔ Fixation on certain numbers

Compulsions involve rituals or various sorts of behaviour that your child feels compelled to repeat over and over. Common childhood compulsions include the following:

- ✔ Arranging objects in a precise manner
- ✔ Excessive hand washing
- ✔ Hoarding items of dubious value
- ✔ Repeatedly counting stairs, wall tiles, and steps taken while walking

Many children perform a few harmless rituals that involve *magical thinking* – thinking they can make something happen by just thinking about it or carrying out superstitious behaviours such as crossing their fingers when wishing for something. For example, they may avoid stepping on pavement cracks. However, any child who shows serious signs of OCD should be taken for professional help. The age of the child when the problem first appears isn't significant; what's important is getting help, because OCD tends not to improve without treatment.

Rare anxieties among children

A few anxiety disorders that occur in adults are occasionally also experienced by children.

- ✔ **Agoraphobia** is often a response to panic and involves avoidance of places or situations in which you feel no escape is readily available.
- ✔ **Panic disorder** involves a sudden onset of intense fearfulness, terror, and physical symptoms. It usually doesn't appear until late adolescence or later.
- ✔ **Post-traumatic stress disorder** is a response to some traumatic event in which the person develops hyper-arousal, intrusive thoughts about the event, and avoidance of any reminders of the event.

See Chapter 2 for more details on all these anxiety disorders. If you notice that your child has any of these anxieties, we recommend seeking professional help via your GP.

Nipping Anxiety in the Bud

How does anxiety begin? The risk for developing anxiety begins at conception. That's right, studies of twins have demonstrated that almost half of what causes anxiety lies in your genes. However, that's just the beginning. Many other factors come into play, and there's a lot you can about it, as we explain.

Understanding early mastery experiences

When a hungry or uncomfortable baby cries out and parents respond by feeding or comforting, the baby has experienced an early sense of *mastery*. In other words, what the baby does results in a predictable, desirable outcome. This early opportunity can then be repeated thousands of times over the next few years in various ways. For example, the toddler discovers how to use language to make requests that then get rewarded. If parents respond unpredictably and chaotically to an infant's attempts to have some control, anxiety is likely to increase.

So in order to decrease the probability of developing anxiety, responding predictably to young children is very important. For young infants, parents should respond with reasonable consistency to most of their distress. Later, predictability is still important but should occur only to age-appropriate distress or requests. In other words, you wouldn't want to reinforce a 2-year-old's temper tantrums by giving in.

As your children grow older, you should provide as many opportunities as possible for them to experience a feeling of mastery. You can do this by

✔ Involving them in sport

✔ Interesting them in hobbies that require some skill

✔ Playing games of skill, such as puzzles or Scrabble

✔ Making sure they have the chance to experience success at school and getting help if they start struggling with their studies

✔ Training them to have good manners and social skills

Fine-tuning emotions

One of the most important tasks of childhood consists of learning how to control emotions, tolerate frustration, and delay gratification. Babies' needs should be met promptly. However, as children grow up, they are expected to stop demanding instant gratification and keep a reasonable lid on their emotional outbursts.

You can help your child learn these crucial skills of emotional control. Helping children express emotions, but not let them run amok, involves a few basic steps:

- **Validate your child's emotions.** When your child feels distressed, anxious, or worried, validate the emotion. You do that by saying,

    'I can see that you are a little scared of . . . '

    'You seem worried about . . . '

    As you can see, this validating statement should also try to help your child connect the feeling to what's going on.

- **Don't deny your children's feelings.** To the greatest degree possible, don't deny the feeling or try to take it away. In other words, you don't want to say, 'You shouldn't be scared', or worse, 'You're not really frightened.'

- **Don't overprotect.** No-one likes to see children feel scared or anxious. However, they need to work out how to deal with most fears on their own. If you try to solve all their problems or keep them from all worries and danger, you're doing more harm than good.

- **Help your children learn to calm down.** You can teach them to take a few slow, deep breaths or count to ten slowly. You can also explain that extreme anxiety and fear will gradually fade.

- **Praise your children.** When they make efforts to overcome anxieties, praise them. However, don't punish them for failing to do so.

- **Don't provide unnecessary reassurance.** Making comments such as 'There's nothing to be afraid of' is unhelpful. Children need to find out how to handle a little stress and anxiety on their own. Don't constantly reassure them or you'll prevent them finding their own solutions, and they'll become more anxious too.

Immunising against anxiety

People can develop phobias about a range of situations, activities, animals, and objects. The following list is shared by children and adults:

- Aeroplanes
- Being alone
- Dogs
- Heights
- Rodents
- Snakes

✔ Spiders and insects

✔ Thunder and lightning

If you want to prevent your children from acquiring one of these common phobias, you can 'vaccinate' them. You do that by helping them safely come into contact with the potentially feared event or object before any fears develop.

Try the following activities:

✔ Take your children to a museum or zoo that offers hands-on experiences with snakes and insects.

✔ Go hill-walking together.

✔ Watch a storm from the safety of your living room. Discuss how lightning and thunder work.

✔ If you don't have a dog or cat of your own, visit friends who do or go to an animal sanctuary, particularly one with puppies and kittens.

Research has proved that this method works. For example, studies have shown that children bitten by dogs don't develop a phobia as readily if they have had positive past experiences with dogs. The more experiences that you provide to your child, the better your child's chances are of growing up without phobias.

For all you somewhat phobic parents, try not to make faces or get too squeamish when you inoculate your children against phobias. Don't say, 'Oooh, how horrible!' Even if you feel nervous, try not to show it.

Anxiety's brain chemistry

Recent research at Columbia University explored the effect of the brain chemical serotonin, which is produced naturally in the human body, on the development of anxiety. Experimenters bred mice that lacked important receptors for serotonin, which left the mice unable to utilise this important neurotransmitter. They found that mice between 5 and 20 days old without the ability to process serotonin showed more signs of anxiety as adults. But when they raised mice with normal serotonin receptors and later depleted the mice of serotonin when they had reached adulthood, the mice didn't develop anxiety.

What does this research have to do with anxious children? It points to the importance of biological factors in the development of anxiety. Even prenatal and early infantile experiences may affect emotional wellbeing long into the future. Perhaps treating childhood anxiety early can help to prevent future problems.

More research is needed to understand how all this works. However, we know that not only do biological interventions (such as medication) affect serotonin levels, but it appears that behavioural strategies, such as those described in this book, also alter brain chemistry in productive ways.

Parenting precautions

A parent can make it more likely that their child will develop an anxiety disorder, or a parent can help to prevent anxiety.

- ✔ **Permissive parents** engage with their children and show concern and caring. But permissive parents hate confrontation, and they can't stand seeing their children get upset. Therefore, they set low expectations for their children, and they don't push them to act maturely or to try new things.

- ✔ **Authoritarian parents** represent the opposite extreme. They demand, direct, and expect instant obedience from their children. They control every detail of their children's lives, making their lives highly structured, and tend to be overly hostile.

The permissive parent and authoritarian parent

Both the permissive and the authoritarian types of parents fuel anxiety in children. The following story is about both types. The mother demonstrates permissive parenting, and the father has an authoritarian style.

Four-year-old **Noreen** screams with terror. Her parents rush into her room to see what's wrong. 'There's a bad man in my room; I saw him', she cries. Noreen's mother hugs her, strokes her hair, and tells her, 'Everything will be okay now that Mummy's here.'

Her dad turns on the light. He checks her wardrobe, looks under her bed and snaps, 'There's nobody here. Just stay in your bed and go to sleep. Don't be such a baby.'

When this happens again, night after night for six weeks in a row, Noreen's dad becomes increasingly annoyed and tells her off for what he calls her silly fears. At the same time, her mother overprotects Noreen. Noreen's mum even starts to sleep in Noreen's room to make her feel safe. Her fears only intensify. Poor Noreen receives mixed messages from her parents, and neither message helps.

Authoritative parenting

A different kind of parenting can help your children deal better with anxiety. It's called *authoritative* parenting (as opposed to authoritarian). Authoritative parents provide clear expectations for their children. They encourage their children to face challenges. They validate their children's feelings of anxiety, but urge them to deal with them. They aren't harsh or punitive, but they don't either criticise or overprotect. Using Noreen's story again, the following demonstrates how authoritative parents would deal with her anxieties.

Four-year-old **Noreen** screams with terror. Her parents rush into her room to see what's wrong. 'There's a bad man in my room; I saw him', she cries.

Noreen's mum gives her a quick hug and says, 'You sound very scared, sweetie.'

Her dad turns on the light, checks the wardrobe, looks under the bed, and says, 'Nobody's here, darling. But if you'd like, we can leave a nightlight on.'

Noreen says, 'No. Can't Mummy just stay here with me tonight?'

Noreen's mum tells her, ''No, it's a much better idea for you learn to go to sleep on your own. I know you're worried, but it will be okay.' They turn the nightlight on, and tell her, 'Here's your bear; he'll keep you company. We'll see you in the morning.'

Noreen cries softly for a few minutes and falls back to sleep.

'But, but, but', you protest, 'I tried that, and it didn't work for me!'

Perhaps your child kept on crying and wouldn't stop. Well, sometimes that happens. Occasionally, you may need to keep up this firm, consistent approach for a few weeks. Eventually, the vast majority of children will fall asleep. And once this starts to happen, the crying is likely to become less and less frequent until it no longer occurs at all. If the crying doesn't stop after a few weeks, you may need to consult a professional.

Helping Already Anxious Children

Perhaps you have anxious children. Don't make yourself anxious by blaming yourself for the problem. Lots of things probably contributed to the development of their anxiety, plus you probably didn't read this book before they developed anxiety, so you didn't know what you could do to prevent it. So what do you do now?

Helping yourself first

Most of you have probably heard the cabin crew's safety briefing on an aeroplane, telling you how to deal with the oxygen masks should they drop down. They tell you to put the mask on yourself before assisting your child. That's because if you don't help yourself first, you won't be in any condition to help your child.

The same principle applies to anxiety in your children. You need to deal with your own anxiety before trying to help your children. Remember, they learn a lot of their emotional responses by observing and copying their parents. It makes sense that anxious parents therefore often have anxious children. The nice part of getting rid of your own anxiety first is that this is likely to help your children. It will also give you the resources to help them with their worries.

This book can both be helpful for you plus enable you to help your children. Pick and choose the strategies that best fit your problem and personality. However, if the ideas you choose first don't seem to work, don't despair. For most people, success is likely when they use one or more of the techniques that we describe.

Modelling mellow

If you don't have a problem with anxiety or if you've largely overcome your excessive worries, you're ready to *model,* or show by example. Children learn a great deal by watching the people they care about. You may remember a time when your child surprised you by repeating words you thought or wished he or she hadn't heard. Trust us, children see and hear everything.

Take advantage of every opportunity to model relatively calm behaviour and thinking. Don't invalidate your child's anxiety by saying it's a stupid or silly fear. Furthermore, demonstrating complete calm is not as useful as showing how you handle the concern yourself. Table 17-2 shows some common child-hood fears and how you can demonstrate an effective response.

Table 17-2	Modelling a Better Way
Fear	*Parental Modelling*
Thunderstorms	I think there's going to be a thunderstorm tonight. Sometimes I find them a bit scary. That's okay, because I know that we're safe at home. If I'm outside, I'll always look for shelter during a thunderstorm. But I know that thunderstorms can't hurt you when you're inside.
Insects	I used to think that insects were horrible and scary, but now I realise that they're more afraid of me than I am of them. Insects run away from people when they can. Sometimes, they're so scared that they freeze. Guess what? I use loads of tissues to pick them up, and that's okay. Let me show you how I do it.
Heights	I sometimes feel a bit scared when I look down from high places. Here we are at the top of the London Eye. Let's hold hands and go to the window together. You can't fall out, and it can't hurt you. Looking down from heights can be fun. It feels kind of exciting after you get used to it.
Being alone (Unnecessary unless your child expressed anxiety about feeling safe alone.)	Dad's on night shift this week. I used to hate being at home on my own. But I worked out that I can look after us both just fine. We've got a burglar alarm, and I always make sure the outside doors and windows are locked. And if anyone did try to get in, we can always call the police. Our dogs are pretty good protection too. Do you ever get scared? If you do, we can talk about it.

Helping children face their fears

As we discuss in Chapter 8, gradual exposure to whatever causes anxiety is one of the most effective ways of overcoming fear. Whether the anxious person is a child or an adult, the strategy is much the same. Therefore, if you want to help your children who already have anxiety, first model coping as we described in Table 17-2 in this chapter. Then consider using *exposure,* which involves tackling the feared situation or object by taking small steps. You gradually confront and stay with each step until anxiety reduces by half or more.

Read Chapter 8 for important additional details about exposure. However, keep a few things in mind when helping your child in this way:

- ✔ **Expect to see some distress.** This is the hard part for parents. No-one likes to see their children get upset. But you can't avoid having your children feel some distress if you want them to get over their anxiety. Sometimes parents find it's too difficult. In this case, a close friend or relative may be willing to help. At the same time, if your child shows extreme anxiety and distress, you need to break the task down further or get professional help.

- ✔ **Praise your child for any successes.** Pay attention to any improvement and compliment your child.

- ✔ **Show patience.** Don't get so overwrought that your own emotions spill over and frighten your child further. Again, if that happens, take a break, enlist a friend's assistance, or seek a professional's advice.

Natalie and Stan, both keen swimmers, plan a dream holiday in the sun. The hotel is right on the beach, and the brochure describes a family-friendly atmosphere. They buy a snorkel and diving mask for their 6-year-old, **David,** who enjoys the plane ride and looks forward to snorkelling with them.

When they arrive, the hotel is as beautiful as promised. The beach beckons, and the water is crystal clear. Natalie, Stan, and David quickly unpack and make their way down to the beach. They walk into the water slowly, delighted by the warm temperature. Suddenly, a large wave breaks in front of them and knocks David over. He opens his mouth in surprise, and salt water chokes him. He cries and runs back to the shore, screaming.

They spend the rest of the holiday unsuccessfully trying to persuade David to go back into the sea. They end up taking turns looking after him, and their dream holiday fades away.

At home, David's fear grows, as untreated fears often do. He fusses in the bath, not wanting any water to splash on his face. He won't even consider getting into a swimming pool.

David's parents take the lead and guide him through exposure. First, on a hot day, they get an inflatable paddling pool, and set it up in the garden. They fill it and model getting in. Eventually, David shows a little interest and joins them in the pool. After he gets more comfortable, the parents do a little playful splashing with each other and encourage David to splash them. He doesn't notice that his own face gets a little water on it.

Then his parents suggest that David put just part of his face into the water. He resists at first, but they encourage him. When he puts his chin into the water, they applaud. Stan bets David that he can't put his whole face in. David proves him wrong.

The parents provide a wide range of gradually increasing challenges, including using the mask and snorkel in pools of various sizes. Eventually, they take another seaside holiday and David learns to love snorkelling.

Relaxing reduces anxiety

Children benefit from learning to relax, much in the same way that adults do. We discussed relaxation methods for adults in Chapters 12 and 13, but children need some slightly different strategies. That's because they don't have the same attention span as adults.

Usually, we suggest teaching children relaxation on an individual basis rather than in groups. Children in groups tend to get embarrassed. They deal with their embarrassment by acting silly and then fail to derive much benefit from the session. Individual sessions don't usually create as much embarrassment, and it's easier to keep children focused.

Breathing relaxation

The following instructions are intended to teach children abdominal breathing, which has been shown to effectively reduce anxiety. Feel free to use your own creativity to design similar instructions.

1. Lie down on the floor and put your hands on your tummy.

2. Pretend that your tummy is a big balloon and that you want to fill it as full as you can.

3. Breathe in and see how big you can make your tummy. Now make a whooshing sound like a balloon losing air as you slowly let the air out. Well done!

4. Let's do it again. Breathe in and fill the balloon. Hold it for a moment and then let the air out of your balloon ever so slowly as you make whooshing sounds.

Repeat this instruction for eight or ten breaths. Tell your children to practise it daily.

Relaxing muscles

A particularly effective way of achieving relaxation is through muscle relaxation. The following instructions may help a child relax. Again, feel free to use your creativity. Have your child tense each muscle group for about ten seconds before relaxing. Then relax for about ten seconds.

1. **Sit down in this chair, close your eyes, and relax.**

2. **Pretend the floor is trying to rise up and that you have to push it back down with your legs and feet. Push, push, push.**

   Okay, now relax your legs and feet. Notice how good that feels.

3. **Uh oh. The floor is starting to rise again. Push it back down.**

   Great! Now relax.

4. **Now tighten your tummy muscles. Make your tummy into a shield of armour; strong like Superman. Hold the muscles in.**

   Excellent! Now relax.

5. **One more time; tighten those tummy muscles into steel. Hold it.**

   Great, now relax and see how nice, warm, and relaxed your tummy feels.

6. **Now, spread your fingers and put your hands together in front of your chest. Squeeze your hands together. Pretend you're squeezing play dough between your hands and make it as squished as you can. Push hard and use your arm muscles too.**

   Okay, now relax. Take a deep breath. Hold it. Now let the air out slowly.

7. **Again, spread your fingers wide, and squish play dough between your hands. Hold it.**

   Great. Now relax.

8. **Pretend you're a turtle. You want to go into your shell. To do that, bring your shoulders way up high and try to touch your ears with your shoulders. Feel your head go down into your shell. Hold it.**

   Okay. Now relax. See how nice, warm, and relaxed your shoulders and neck feel.

9. **One more time now. Be a turtle and go into your shell. Hold it.**

   Good. Now relax.

10. **Finally, screw your face up like you do when you eat something that tastes really, really awful. Screw it right up. Really tight. Hold it.**

    Okay; now relax. Take a deep breath. Hold it; now let the air out slowly.

11. One more time. Screw your face up as tight as you can. Hold it.

Relax. Well done! See how limp and relaxed your body feels. If you feel upset or worried, you can do this all by yourself to feel better. You don't have to do all the muscles like we did. You can just do what you want to.

Imagining your way to relaxation

One way to help your child relax is through reading books. Before bed, children find stories very relaxing. Reading gets rid of worries and concerns from the day. You can also find various books, CDs, and tapes specifically designed for helping children relax. Unfortunately, some of these use imagery of beautiful, relaxing scenes that children may find rather boring.

Rather than idyllic scenes of beaches and lakes, children can relax quite nicely to their own fantasies. The scenes don't need be about relaxation as such, they just need to be entertaining and pleasant. Again, the point is to provide engaging alternatives to worries and fears. One great idea was suggested by a child and her mother who came for help. They suggested designing your own book with your child, as they did. The child wrote and illustrated each page of her own relaxation book titled *Imagine Unicorns and Smiling Stars:*

Close your eyes and relax.

Imagine unicorns dancing.

Imagine outer space. Look at the planets spinning and floating.

Imagine smiling stars. See how happy they are.

Imagine blue moons. See the moons smiling.

Imagine nice aliens. They like you.

Imagine spaceships soaring.

Imagine unicorns dancing in outer space with smiling stars, blue moons, and friendly aliens in their spaceship soaring.

Now relax. Dream wonderful dreams.

Exorcising anxiety through exercise

Exercise burns off excess adrenaline, which can otherwise fuel anxiety. All children obviously need regular exercise, and studies show that most don't exercise enough. Anxious children may be reluctant to participate in organised sports. They may feel inadequate or even afraid of how others will see and judge them.

Yet it may be important for anxious children to participate in sports for two reasons. First, sports can provide them with important mastery experiences. Although they may feel frustrated and upset at first, they usually experience considerable pride and a sense of achievement as their skills improve. Secondly, aerobic activity directly decreases anxiety.

The challenge is to find a sport that provides your child with the greatest possible chance of at least some success. Consider the following activities for your child:

- **Football:** Children burn off a lot of energy in this game. They also learn about teamwork and strategy.

- **Swimming teams:** This is a sport that doesn't involve balls thrown at your head or collisions with other players. Swimmers compete against themselves, and many swimming teams reward most members with ribbons, whether they come first or sixth.

- **Athletics:** This also is an individual sport that has a wide variety of different skill possibilities. Some children are fast and can run short dashes. Others discover that they can develop the endurance to run long distances. Still others can throw a javelin or a shot put.

- **Tennis, table tennis and badminton:** These are low contact and relatively safe sports. Good instruction can make most able-bodied children adequate players.

- **Martial arts:** Good for enhancing a sense of competence and confidence. Many martial arts instructors have great skill for working with uncoordinated, fearful children. Almost all children can experience improvements and success with martial arts.

- **Dance:** This sport includes many different types of dance from traditional dances of different cultures to ballet, jazz, hip hop and street dancing. Musically inclined children often do quite well with dance classes.

Find something for your children to do that involves physical activity. They can benefit in terms of decreased anxiety, increased confidence, and greater interaction with others. Don't forget to include family bike rides and country walks. Model the benefits of lifelong activity and exercise.

Chapter 18

Coping with Your Partner's Anxiety

*E*ven people who live together sometimes don't know each other as well as they think they do. That's because many people try not to show any signs of what they consider are weaknesses, limitations, and vulnerability.

This chapter helps you communicate with your partner at times when he or she experiences anxiety. With the right communication style, rather than stirring up anger and resentment, you can take on a different, helpful role. You can also combine forces to tackle anxiety by finding ways to simplify life, have fun, and relax together. Finally, find out how simply accepting your partner's anxiety and limitations can lead to a better relationship and, paradoxically, to less anxiety.

Discovering Whether Your Partner Suffers with Anxiety

Why do people hide their anxious feelings? Fear and upbringing are two big reasons:

✔ Revealing negative feelings can be embarrassing, especially for someone with an anxiety disorder. People are often reluctant to admit to experiencing anxiety, because they often fear rejection or ridicule. However, in practice, admitting feelings is usually helpful and also brings people closer together.

✔ Children may have been taught to hide or deny feelings by their parents. They may have been told, 'Don't be such a baby', or, 'Boys don't cry.' When that happens, they often grow up having learned to keep their worries to themselves. If we are encouraged to express feelings earlier in life, it makes it much easier to do so when we are adults, rather than having to learn this later in life, perhaps after things have gone wrong for us.

So how do you really know whether your partner has a problem with anxiety? And does it matter whether you know? We think that it does matter. Knowing whether your partner experiences anxiety can lead to better understanding and communication between the two of you.

The following list may help you to identify whether your partner suffers from anxiety. Ask yourself whether your partner:

✔ Seems restless and on edge?

✔ Avoids situations for seemingly trivial reasons?

✔ Is preoccupied, worrying about future catastrophes?

✔ Is reluctant to leave the house?

✔ Has trouble sleeping?

✔ Has trouble concentrating?

✔ Is plagued with self-doubts?

✔ Is constantly on the alert for dangers?

✔ Worries excessively about germs, contamination, or dirt?

✔ Frequently re-checks such things as whether the doors are locked, windows closed, or that the cooker is switched off?

✔ Seems terrified by specific things, such as insects, dogs, thunderstorms, and so on?

✔ Responds with irritation when pushed to attend social functions, such as parties, weddings, meetings, and work functions?

Note: The resistance may be due to simple dislike of the activity, but carefully consider whether anxiety may be at the root of the problem.

Some of the symptoms in the preceding list (especially irritability, poor concentration, poor sleep, and self-doubts) may also indicate depression. Depression is a serious condition that usually also includes loss of interest in activities previously considered pleasurable, change in appetite, and depressed mood. See Chapter 2 for more information about depression. If your partner seems depressed, talk with them and then consult with a mental health practitioner or your family doctor.

If you answered yes to any of the questions in the preceding list (and your partner doesn't seem particularly depressed), we don't recommend that you approach your partner and say, 'Look at this list. Now I know what's the matter with you!' This probably wouldn't be very helpful at all.

Instead, consider asking your partner a few questions. Don't do so just after a disagreement or an argument. Ways to approach the subject include:

- ✔ You've seemed a bit on edge lately. What's been bothering you?
- ✔ What's the most stressful thing for you at the moment?
- ✔ What's worrying you the most?
- ✔ Sometimes, when I go to events like this, I feel anxious. I wonder how you feel about going?
- ✔ I noticed you've had trouble sleeping lately. What's been on your mind?

Try to make your questions as non-threatening and safe to answer as possible. In addition, think about asking questions that don't have a simple yes or no answer. For example, if you ask your partner whether he or she is anxious, the reply may be a simple 'No', and then the discussion is over.

The quiz about your partner's anxiety and the suggestions of how to broach the subject can enable you both to start talking about anxiety. After you confirm that your partner is struggling with anxiety, you can develop a plan together to deal with it. But you need to know how to build on the initial discussion.

Talking Together about Anxiety

Talking about a partner's vulnerability isn't always easy. Keeping a few ideas in mind may help. For example, if you find the conversation turning into an argument, leave it alone for now. Your partner may not be ready to face the problem. If so, check out the 'Accepting Anxiety with Love' section, later in this chapter.

Not every couple can communicate easily about difficult subjects without arguing. If that's the case for the two of you, we suggest relationship counselling because reading a few pages about talking together won't solve fundamental communication problems. However, as a couple, if you're able to talk about anxiety without experiencing a breakdown in communication, we have some general guidelines for you.

Sometimes, one person in a relationship actually prefers to take care of the other or even feels more powerful knowing that the other has a problem. Such a partner may sabotage, rather than assist, the other's efforts to deal with the problem. If your partner starts to sabotage your efforts, seek relationship counselling or individual therapy.

Helping, not taking over responsibility

The first requirement in any discussion of your partner's anxiety is to show *empathic concern*. That means putting yourself in your partner's shoes and seeing the world from your partner's point of view. Then you can try to understand the source of the worry.

However, expressing empathy and concern doesn't mean that you need to solve the problem. You can't. You may be able to help, as we show in the 'Guiding the Way' section later in this chapter, but you don't control other people's emotions – that's their own responsibility.

It's important to realise that helpers don't own the responsibility for making change happen. Unless you accept this, you're likely to become frustrated and angry if and when efforts to change get stuck. Frustration and anger only make overcoming anxiety more difficult.

Avoiding blame

While you shouldn't blame yourself by owning the problem when your partner becomes anxious, it's equally important to avoid blaming your partner. Your partner developed anxiety for all the reasons we list in Chapter 3. Nobody asks for an anxiety disorder. Nobody wants one, and change is difficult.

People are particularly tempted to blame their partners if they make great efforts to help, yet their partners seem ungrateful and resistant. You must understand that anxiety's tentacles tenaciously tighten their grip when threatened. That's because anxiety's like an old habit. It may not feel good, but at least it's familiar. When you start to work on reducing anxiety, anxiety typically increases before it decreases and you overcome it.

Do make every effort to avoid blame and, above all, be patient. Success and failure aren't up to you. You want to help, but if change doesn't happen, that's certainly not your fault, and isn't because you weren't sufficiently helpful.

When help turns into harm

People with anxiety desperately seek ways to alleviate their distress. One common way is to ask for reassurance. If your partner has anxiety, of course you want to help by giving that reassurance. For example, people who have a great fear of illness often ask their partner if they look unwell or if they're running a temperature. Reassuring your partner presents one problem – it makes matters worse.

How can something intended to alleviate anxiety create more? Well, the immediate reduction in anxiety reinforces or rewards the act of seeking assistance. Thus, rather than learning to depend on one's own good sense, giving reassurance teaches the other person to look for answers elsewhere. Both dependency and anxiety thereby increase. Here's an example of how reassurance can aggravate anxiety.

James and **Roberto** are first year students at a famous College of Music. They have decided to live together and they lead busy lives. With all the pressure of rehearsals and academic work, James has recently stopped attending social events, complaining of tiredness. Roberto has found himself going alone.

Last year, Roberto received a major music award for being an outstanding young musician. He is invited to perform and to receive the award at a prestigious concert hall in London. Of course, he wants James to attend, but James is scared of sitting alone and feeling trapped. Roberto reassures James that the auditorium is safe and that he could get out if he needed to by booking an aisle seat, and that he doesn't have to take one of the music college's complimentary tickets. James still resists, so Roberto suggests they could buy another ticket for a friend to attend and keep James company whilst Roberto is performing.

Finally, after considerable cajoling, reassurance, and extra measures to ensure his comfort, James's worries about feeling trapped decrease and he agrees to go to the concert. However, as the evening progresses, James seems to need increasingly more reassurance and attention. He withdraws more and his anxiety increases. At the interval, he says that he is feeling unwell and leaves, missing Roberto's performance despite all that has been put in place to help. Roberto feels both rejected and absolutely gutted.

What can we learn from this story? Roberto made the mistake of not only being empathetic but also of trying to own James's problem. Unfortunately, when you try to take on your partner's problem as your own, by giving too much reassurance and excessive help, it usually makes things worse. Dependency, avoidance, and anxiousness all increase. It's a matter of balance. Give truly needed help, show real concern, but avoid going too far.

If you've been in the habit of giving your partner frequent large doses of re-assurance, don't suddenly stop without discussing the issue first. Otherwise, your partner is likely to think that you've stopped caring. You need to let your partner know and come to an agreement that eliminating unnecessary reassurance is a good idea. Then agree that you will reassure once on any given concern, but when asked repeatedly, you will simply smile and say, 'We agreed that I can't answer that.'

Guiding the Way

Assuming you've had a helpful, productive discussion with your partner about the anxiety problem, you may be able to help even more. But first, take a look at yourself. If you also wrestle with anxiety, do all that you can to help yourself before trying to tackle your partner's anxiety.

Only after you've dealt with your own anxiety should you consider helping your partner overcome theirs. You'll need to provide encouragement, help develop plans, show what's not working, and also provide support. Part of your job is to model how to handle stress and worry. You can't do a good job of modelling if you're quaking in your boots.

You can help plan and direct using one of the most effective ways of overcoming anxiety: gradual exposure. *Exposure* involves breaking down any given fear into small steps and facing it. Most importantly, exposure asks the person to stay with each step until the anxiety has reduced by at least half. If any given step creates too much anxiety, you can help devise ways of breaking the task into even smaller stages.

Be sure to read Chapter 8 for important details about exposure, prior to attempting to help your partner develop an exposure plan. If you run into any difficulty in terms of your partner resisting or arguing with you, consult a professional. Of course you want to help, but it isn't worth harming your relationship to do so. Consider the story of Doug and Rosie.

Doug and **Rosie** have being going out together for over a year. In all that time, they've never gone to the cinema together, because Rosie suffers from agoraphobia. Although she's able to go to most places and do what she needs to in life, she dreads going anywhere that makes her feel trapped, especially the cinema and the theatre. She fantasises that she'll need to get out but she won't find her way to an exit because of the crowd and the darkness. She imagines that she would trip over people, fall on her face, and desperately crawl through the darkened cinema.

Doug realises that Rosie makes one excuse after another to avoid going to the cinema, even though she enjoys watching films on television. Gently, he asks Rosie, 'Some things make me a little anxious – heavy traffic and really large crowds. What makes you anxious?' Rosie confesses that crowded cinemas make her feel closed in and trapped.

Several days later, Doug sees a copy of *Overcoming Anxiety For Dummies* in a bookshop and buys it with Rosie in mind. He starts reading, paying particular attention to Chapter 8 about exposure. Doug and Rosie have a productive discussion about Rosie's concerns and decide it's time to face them. Doug volunteers to help support Rosie through the process.

First, they jointly devise a tower of fear, which breaks down the feared situation into small steps. (See more on the tower of fear in Chapter 8.) Rosie's tower of fear consists of ten blocks. Figure 18-1 shows five of Rosie's blocks.

Doug has a role to play in most of Rosie's tasks. Not only does he accompany her, he celebrates her successes and encourages her to persist when she starts to falter. He holds her hand on the earlier items and needs to give less support towards the end. Rosie needs to go to several films with Doug before she agrees to her final task of going on her own.

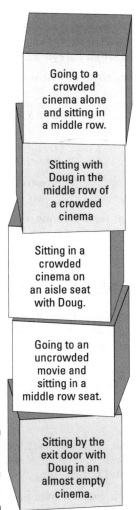

Figure 18-1:
Rosie's tower of fear.

Going to a crowded cinema alone and sitting in a middle row.

Sitting with Doug in the middle row of a crowded cinema

Sitting in a crowded cinema on an aisle seat with Doug.

Going to an uncrowded movie and sitting in a middle row seat.

Sitting by the exit door with Doug in an almost empty cinema.

Rosie and Doug go to the cinema complex together on when Rosie deals with the last item in her tower of fear, but he chooses the film playing on a different screen. Although Rosie feels frightened, she stays with her film, and sticks it out. She feels delighted with her achievement, and the two of them become closer.

So just exactly how do you help your partner?

✔ Begin only if your partner clearly expresses an interest and a desire for your assistance. It won't work if your partner doesn't want to change or to have you involved.

✔ Define your role. In other words, come to a clear understanding of how much and what input your partner wants from you. Would your partner like you to be involved in the planning? In what way? Does your partner want to be accompanied and encouraged when carrying out the plan?

• Ask whether your partner wants you to simply observe or actively encourage.

• Ask whether you should hold hands, stand next to your partner, or stand a few feet away.

✔ Help your partner develop the plan, but don't take on the full responsibility for designing the exposure hierarchy. (See Chapter 8 for details.)

✔ Keep your own emotions in check. Don't let your desire to help overwhelm you and cause you to help excessively.

✔ Don't let your emotions cause you to push your partner too much. Respect your partner's decisions to move ahead or not. Give encouragement, but do so gently.

✔ After the plan is in place, expect your partner to have ups and downs. Some days go better than others. Remember, determining how the plan works out in practice isn't up to you.

✔ Before asking your partner to carry out a step, offer to model the task first. If you model, showing a small amount of anxiety yourself, if you really feel it, is fine. Just don't try to model actions that you personally can't do.

✔ Practice going through the steps with imagery first. Don't carry it out in real life until your partner feels more comfortable with the imagery. You can consult Chapter 8 for details about how to use your imagination as well.

✔ Set up some rewards for success at various stages in the hierarchy. Do something you both can enjoy together. You can also give some honest praise for success; just be sure not to sound patronising.

✔ If your partner appears anxious at any step, but not overwhelmed, encourage your partner to stay with that step until the anxiety comes down by half. Obviously, don't absolutely insist, just encourage. Remind your partner that anxiety will normally decrease if you just hang on in there for long enough.

It Takes Two: Two Heads Are Better Than One

Another way that you can help your partner overcome anxiety is to collaborate on ways to decrease stress in both of your lives. With a little ingenuity, you can explore a variety of solutions that are likely to feel good to you even if you personally don't suffer from anxiety at all. For example:

- ✔ **Take a stress management class at a local adult education centre.** These classes help people make lifestyle changes and set goals. Many of the ideas make life more fun and interesting in addition to reducing stress.

- ✔ **Take regular walks with your partner.** It's a great way to reduce stress, but even if you don't have much stress, strolling under the sky together offers a wonderful time to talk and is great for your health.

- ✔ **Take a yoga class together.** Again, even if you don't have anxiety, yoga is terrific for balance, muscle strength, flexibility, and overall health.

- ✔ **Explore spirituality together.** You may choose to attend a church, synagogue, mosque, or temple, or explore less traditional methods of communing with a higher power, such as immersing yourselves in nature. Thinking about things bigger than yourselves or even the mundane events of the world provides a peaceful perspective.

- ✔ **Look for creative ways to simplify your joint lives.** Consider looking for help with household chores if you both work. Carefully analyse the way that you spend time and make sure that your time reflects your priorities. See Chapter 9 for more ideas.

- ✔ **Get away.** Take a holiday. You don't have to spend much money. And if you don't have the time for a long break, go away for an occasional one- or two-night weekend getaway. Getting away from the telephone, computer, doorbell, and the endless tasks and demands, even for a night, can help rejuvenate you both.

Accepting Anxiety with Love

It may seem rather counter-intuitive, but accepting your partner's battle with anxiety is one of the most useful attitudes that you can take. Acceptance paradoxically forms the foundation for change. In other words, whenever you discuss your partner's anxiety or engage in any effort to help, you need to appreciate and love all your partner's strengths and weaknesses.

You fell in love with the whole package – not just the good stuff. After all, you're not perfect and nor is your partner. You wouldn't want perfection if you had it. If perfect people even existed, we can only imagine that they would be quite boring. Besides, studies show that people who try to be perfect more often become depressed, anxious, and distressed.

Therefore, rather than expecting perfection, accept your loved one 'as is'. You need to accept and embrace both the possibility of productive change as well as the chance that your partner may remain stuck. Accepting your partner is especially important when your efforts to help:

- ✔ Result in an argument
- ✔ Seem ineffective
- ✔ Are not well received by your partner
- ✔ Seem merely to increase your partner's anxiety even after repeated efforts at exposure

What does acceptance do? More than you may think. Acceptance allows partners to join together and grow closer, because acceptance avoids putting pressure on your partner. Intense expectations only serve to increase anxiety and resistance to change.

Acceptance conveys the message that you will love your partner no matter what. You still care, whether your partner stays the same or succeeds in making changes. This message frees your partner to

- ✔ Take risks
- ✔ Make mistakes
- ✔ Feel vulnerable
- ✔ Feel loved

Change requires risk-taking, vulnerability, and mistakes. When people feel that they can safely get things wrong, look silly, cry, or fail miserably, they can take those risks. Think about it. When do you take risks or try new things? Probably not when you're near a critical audience.

Overcoming anxiety and fear takes tremendous courage in order to face the risks involved. Letting go of your need to see your partner change helps bolster the courage your partner needs. Letting go of your need includes giving up ego. In other words, this is not about you.

When you take on the role of a helper, it doesn't mean that your worth is at stake. Of course, you want to do the best you can, but you can't force others to change. Your partner ultimately must own the responsibility.

Part VI
The Part of Tens

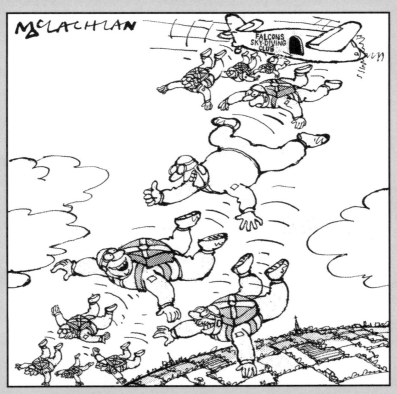

'Took ages to persuade Darren to come sky diving. He was always anxious about whether his parachute would open or not.'

In this part . . .

We offer ten quick ways to defeat anxious feelings on the spot. Discover ten strategies that may look like ways to deal with anxiety but that just don't work. If anxiety comes back, we review ten ways of dealing with such relapses. Also, be sure to take a look at the ten indications that you may need professional help.

Chapter 19

Ten Ways to Stop Anxiety Quickly

Sometimes you need quick, temporary relief from anxiety. With that in mind, this chapter describes ten handy techniques to use when worry and stress start getting out of hand.

Breathing Out Your Anxiety

Anxiety tends to make breathing shallow and rapid, which in turn increases anxiety – a vicious circle. Try this quick, easy-to-learn breathing technique to restore a calming pattern of breathing. You can do this any time, anywhere. It really works. Give it a try.

1. Breathe in deeply through your nose.

2. Hold your breath for a few seconds.

3. Slowly let your breath out through your lips while making a slight sound, such as hissing or sighing.

4. Repeat Steps 1 to 3 for a minimum of ten breaths.

Talking with a Friend

Anxiety is a lonely feeling, and loneliness increases anxiety. Research shows that social support helps people deal better with almost any type of emotional distress. So don't hesitate to reach out to friends and family. Confide in someone you trust. You may think that no-one wants to hear about your troubles, but we're not talking about whining and complaining. We're talking about sharing what you're going through and where you're at.

No doubt you would do the same for someone else. People exist to turn to in troubled times. If you find yourself without friends, consider speaking to someone such as a minister, priest, imam or rabbi. If you don't take part in formal religion, call a help line. You can also see Chapter 22 for signs that you may need professional help, and if you do, where to find it.

Exercising Aerobically

Anxiety usually floods the body with adrenaline. Adrenaline makes your heart beat faster and your muscles tighten and causes various other body sensations that feel distressing. Nothing burns off adrenaline faster than aerobic exercise. See Chapter 10 for more information about this. Good examples include: jogging; a long, fast walk; dancing; skipping; and badminton.

Soothing the Body

One of the most distressing aspects of anxiety is that it makes your body feel tense, queasy, and shaky. Quick ways to temporarily break through the tension include the following:

- ✔ Soaking in a hot bath for a good while.
- ✔ Taking a long hot shower.
- ✔ Enjoying a 15-minute massage, either from a masseur or using a mat with an electronic heating and vibrating massager.

Taking Rescue Remedy

Rescue Remedy is one of a series of remedies derived from flowers and is available from health shops and mainstream chemists and pharmacists. A few drops on your tongue or added to water and sipped slowly can provide rapid relief. However, do check with your doctor before taking any herbal remedies because of possible interactions with other drugs.

Challenging Your Anxious Thinking

The way you think strongly influences the way you feel. Anxious people inevitably think about things in ways that increase their anxiety. One of the best ways of dealing with anxiety is to examine the evidence supporting your anxious thoughts.

First, write down what you're worried about. Afterwards, ask yourself some questions about those thoughts, such as

- ✔ Is this really as bad as I think?
- ✔ Can some evidence contradict my anxious thoughts?
- ✔ In a year from now, how important will this event be to me?
- ✔ Am I making a dire prediction without any real basis?

After answering these questions, try to write down a more realistic perspective. See Chapter 5 to discover more about how to write out your anxious thoughts, analyse them for distortions, and replace them with more realistic, calmer thoughts.

Listening to Music

Sounds influence the way that you feel. Think about it. If you listen to fingernails scraping across a blackboard, how do you feel? Most people report that it gives them a crawling, shuddering, anxious feeling. Just as unpleasant sounds jangle the nerves, soothing sounds can calm you.

Select music that you find relaxing. Get comfortable and close your eyes. Turn the volume to a comfortable level. Relax. Listen.

Alternative Activities

Avoiding your anxiety isn't a good idea. But until you discover more direct ways of tackling it, it can be useful to get absorbed in other activities. Consider the following:

- ✔ A good book
- ✔ A film

> ✔ Television
>
> ✔ Computer games
>
> ✔ Indulging yourself!

Making Love

If you have an available, willing partner, sex is a wonderful way to relax. It can certainly take your mind off anxiety! And, like aerobic exercise, it burns off adrenalin. What a perfect combination.

Some anxious people get very worried about their sexual performance. If that's you, don't try this strategy until you overcome your anxiety about this issue. And, if you don't have an available, willing partner, we don't recommend hiring one.

Staying with the Moment

What are you worried about? Chances are, it's something that hasn't even happened yet and may never occur. The fact is, almost 90 per cent of what people worry about never actually happens. And if it does occur, it rarely ends up as catastrophic as the worriers predict.

Therefore, we suggest that you focus on the here and now. What are you doing? Look around you. Notice how the air feels as you breathe in and out. Feel your feet and the muscles in your legs as you sit. If you still feel anxiety, study it. Notice the various sensations in your body and realise that they won't kill you. They pass eventually, even as you are observing them. If you accept that you're feeling just a bit anxious, the feelings pass more quickly than if you tell yourself that you must get rid of them at once. Read Chapter 16 for more ideas about mindful acceptance.

Enjoy the moment.

Chapter 20

Ten Anxiety Busters
That Just Don't Work

*M*ost of this book gives you ideas for how to deal with anxiety. This chapter tells you what not to do. Don't feel bad if you've previously tried one or more of these ways of coping with your anxiety. Some are indeed tempting. But research studies and clinical experience tell us that they just don't work and may even make anxiety worse.

Avoiding What Scares You

Why not? If you're afraid of snakes, it's perfectly natural to stay away from them. Or if you worry about driving on motorways, why not stick to A and B roads? The problem with avoidance is that it feels too good. Staying away becomes a pattern. *Avoidance feeds anxiety.*

That's because people with high levels of anxiety can feel nervous about many things. After they avoid one thing, another fear often develops. Avoidance worked for the first one, so why not avoid this one too? Eventually, fears, like weeds, choke and crowd out a healthy life. Furthermore, behaviour influences your beliefs. Avoidance behaviour also increases fear because it feeds your belief that what you're avoiding is seriously scary. For example, **Alan** felt uncomfortable in crowds. He worried about not being able to escape from stadiums if he felt the need. So he avoided sporting events. That worked pretty well, but then he noticed he was anxious in crowded shopping centres. So he let his wife do most of the shopping. No big deal. But then he started to feel uncomfortable in restaurants. And so on . . .

Whining and Complaining

'Why me?'

'It isn't fair.'

'I hate being anxious. I can't stand it.'

People with these attitudes hope others will rescue them. They complain constantly and do little to help themselves. Some even seem to get something out of complaining, while others look for sympathy.

But that doesn't work. People don't like being bombarded with endless negativity. It only puts people off. Overcoming anxiety takes work and commitment. Not whining and complaining.

 We're not talking about just discussing and sharing your problems with a friend or loved one here. Sharing your concerns can be a useful way to reduce your anxiety and obtain a little support. What's the difference between sharing and complaining? Whiners usually drone on and on and have little interest in exploring productive solutions. They usually respond to each possibility by saying 'Yes, but . . .' and then continue at length about how they've tried that already and it didn't work, or assure you it won't work because . . .

Seeking Reassurance

'Please come to town with me.'

'Do I look like I'm coming down with something?'

Like the whiners and complainers, some people look to others to solve their problems. They want constant help and reassurance from their friends, families, and colleagues. Instead of facing their fears on their own, they lean on others and become dependent.

It's fine to look to others when you really need help, but when you continuously ask for reassurance, you're not dealing with your own worries. The reassurance only works temporarily. It does reduce anxiety for the moment, but problem is that it also reinforces the belief that you can't handle things on your own, which makes you even more anxious in the longer term.

Wishing and Hoping

How nice life would be if that fancy bottle really held a genie just waiting to grant all your wishes. Just rub the bottle and whoosh, a genie appears to instantly banish all your anxiety, worry, and stress. Nice thought. But miracles seldom happen.

Nothing is wrong with hope. People need hope. However, hope on its own is unlikely to be sufficient to make the changes you want to your life. Hope combined with dedicated effort can start you on the road to recovery.

Looking for a Quick Fix

'Get rid of your anxiety in three hours!'

'Listen to these tapes and never feel anxious again; just £24.99.'

'Take advantage of our one-day-only special offer and get free postage and packaging!'

That sounds great. But like most quick fixes, if it sounds too good to be true, it probably is. Instant cures usually enrich the seller at the buyer's expense. Be guided by research when choosing your solutions.

Drowning Your Anxiety

I tried to drown my anxiety, but it learned to swim!

Many people turn to alcohol to calm down. And in the short run, let's face it; it can feel like it helps. After work, relaxing with a drink can feel pretty good. In fact, research suggests that for healthy adults, drinking some alcohol, for instance wine, may even have a few health benefits. So what's wrong with drinking to relax?

✔ Drinking can become a habit.

✔ You may need more and more to feel an effect.

✔ Drinking disrupts sleep.

✔ Alcohol is highly calorific.

✔ Alcohol impairs co-ordination.

✔ Drinking can prevent you from dealing with your problems.

So if the occasional glass of wine or pint of beer is what you enjoy, it's unlikely to harm you. But if your consumption substantially increases, watch out, you probably have a problem.

Eating for Comfort

When you've got anxiety gnawing away in the pit of your stomach, it can be all too easy to try to fill that hungry, empty feeling by eating something – preferably something fatty, starchy, or sugary. Then, as you put on weight, you'll probably get anxious about that, in addition to whatever else was initially worrying you. You may start feeling tired and depressed. Try to discriminate between pangs of hunger and pangs of anxiety. If you think that the cause is anxiety, see what alternatives you have to eating. Just as you can't drown your anxiety, neither does feeding it with calories make it go away.

Trying Too Hard

Extreme measures rarely work. Just like wishing without putting any effort in to overcome anxiety doesn't work, trying *too* hard is likely to backfire. Why? Because being anxious about being anxious can make you really anxious! Think about it. If you absolutely *must* get rid of your anxiety, you become anxious about doing everything right.

Let's face it; you've had your anxiety for a long time. It takes time to reduce it, and you'll never reach a point when anxiety goes away completely unless you're dead or in a coma. Be realistic and patient. Make progress; don't expect perfection.

Keeping a Stiff Upper Lip

The British are renowned for keeping a lid on their feelings. But like a pressure cooker, if things start to boil, and the steam can't escape, watch out because it's likely to explode.

Taking Medication as the Sole Solution

Chapter 15 discusses the medication used in the treatment of anxiety. Yet we now seem to be saying that medications don't work. Actually, that's not the case. *Medication works extremely well for some people.* However, many people can't tolerate the side effects; others don't want to take pills. Some worry about the long-term effects of medication. Most importantly, medication doesn't teach people how to draw on their own resources to deal with their problems.

One class of drugs, the benzodiazepines, can sometimes interfere with the long-term benefits of exposure therapy. Although benzodiazepines are helpful in selected cases, they can also be addictive.

However, certain medication can provide relief. Pills alone just aren't the magical cure that many hope for.

Chapter 21

Ten Ways to Deal with Relapse

*I*f you're reading this chapter, you've probably made some headway with your anxiety. But maybe, after all your hard work, you've experienced a setback or are worried about having one. Don't panic! We have ten strategies you can use when anxiety knocks on your door.

Expecting Anxiety

Perhaps you've worked hard to overcome your anxiety. And now your hard work has paid off. You've beaten it. Congratulations! But horror of horrors, one day you wake up and suddenly discover anxiety staring you in the face. You turn it into a catastrophe and assume that you've failed.

Come off it! You'll never totally annihilate anxiety. That is, until you stop breathing. It's bound to show up from time to time. Expect anxiety. Look for its early warning signs. But don't make things worse by getting anxious about your anxiety. If you understand that anxiety will return, you can reduce its impact.

Understanding That Relapses Pass Too

Anxiety has an ebb and flow. The proverb 'One swallow doesn't make a summer' reflects the fact that a single sign doesn't necessarily indicate that something more is inevitable. Just because you have an anxious episode or two doesn't mean that you're back to square one. You worked out how to deal with your anxiety before, and that knowledge can still help you. You don't need to start all over again when anxiety returns.

You need to move forward and reapply what you've already practised. Don't make a crisis out of a problem. Catastrophising about minor setbacks will only increase your anxiety and immobilise your efforts. Regroup, reorganise, and get back on track!

Finding Out Why Anxiety Returned

Minor relapses are a great opportunity to discover what triggers your anxiety. Work out what was happening just before your latest bout of anxiety:

- ✔ Have you had some recent difficulties at work, such as deadlines, promotions, problems with colleagues, and the like?
- ✔ Have you had recent problems at home?
- ✔ Have you experienced some major life changes, such as marriage, divorce, the birth of a child, financial setbacks, or a loss of some sort?

It's useful to be aware that an increase in your anxiety is a natural response to some events and likely to be temporary. Use the new information about your anxiety triggers to challenge your anxious thinking as described in Chapter 5.

Seeing a Doctor

If you looked, and you really can't identify anything that may have triggered the return of your anxiety, consider making an appointment with your doctor. Anxiety can have a number of physical causes:

- ✔ Prescribed medication side effects
- ✔ Over-the-counter medication side effects
- ✔ Dietary supplement side effects
- ✔ Too much caffeine
- ✔ Physical disorders (see Chapter 2)

Don't try to self-diagnose. If you experience anxiety with absolutely no discernable cause, do have a complete physical checkup.

Trying What Worked Before

If anxiety reappears, review the strategies that worked for you previously. Some of these techniques may need to become lifelong habits. Make relaxation (see Chapters 12 and 13) a part of your life. Exercise on a regular basis (see Chapter 10). Make a long-term habit of writing down at least a few of your anxious thoughts and then challenge them (see Chapter 5). Look at your core beliefs now and again and argue with them (see Chapter 6). Are you using too many worry words (see Chapter 7)?

Anxiety isn't a disease that you can cure with a one-time injection, pill, or surgery. Some anxiety is a natural part of life. When it expands to a distressing degree, you merely need to reapply your strategies for dealing with it, and it will contract once again to manageable proportions.

Doing Something Different

We've presented a huge range of strategies for overcoming anxiety. You probably picked a few that felt compatible with your lifestyle. Now consider looking at some you haven't tried yet. Do something different! Take a look at the list that follows and choose one you've not had a go at:

- ✔ Rethinking your anxiety (see Chapters 5, 6, and 7)
- ✔ Facing fear head on (see Chapter 8)
- ✔ Exercise (see Chapter 10)
- ✔ Relaxation strategies (see Chapter 12)

If you've simply dabbled with one or more of these techniques, try it wholeheartedly and see whether that works better. It really is worth considering any you haven't tried yet.

Getting Support

You don't have to face anxiety relapses alone. Talking with others helps you deal with emotional distress. A lot of support groups exist. Try your local library for a list of them.

But what if you live in a small rural village, with no easily accessible support group? All is not lost. You can go to an Internet search engine, such as Google (www.google.com) and enter 'chat rooms for anxiety'. You'll find more than enough interesting sources of support. Try a few out and see whether you can find a group that feels compatible. Millions of people suffer from anxiety, and they have great advice and support to offer you. You don't need to suffer alone. However, be careful of some of the 'self-help' sites that are of the 'self-illness' variety, where people try to compete by being more anxious than everyone else and proclaiming how totally un-helpable they are.

Considering a Top Up

If you've seen a professional and later experienced an unexpected increase in your anxiety, think about requesting a top up of a few more sessions. Your therapist isn't going to think that you've failed. Usually, some further therapy helps and doesn't take as long as before. In addition, some people like to arrange a longer term follow-up, some months ahead, as relapse prevention. Remember, anxiety isn't a disease and there's no magic cure.

On the other hand, if you have never seen a professional, and you experience a relapse, you should consider it now. If you've had previous success on your own, you're likely to improve rapidly with a little assistance.

Looking at the Stages of Change

Any kind of change involves a series of steps or stages. These stages don't necessarily occur in a linear fashion. As discussed in greater detail in Chapter 2, these stages include

- ✔ **Pre-contemplation:** Not even thinking about change. Obviously, you're not at this stage if you're reading this book.
- ✔ **Contemplation:** Thinking about change, but not being ready to do something about it.
- ✔ **Preparation:** Making plans to do something about your problem.
- ✔ **Action:** Meeting the problem head on.
- ✔ **Maintenance:** Making continued efforts to deal with your problem.
- ✔ **Termination:** You no longer even have to think about your problem.

Relapse can occur during any of these stages. For example, you may move back from action to contemplation or even pre-contemplation. Just remember, it's normal. When you step back for a while, it doesn't mean that you can't gather your resources to have another go. Most who succeed have tried a number of times before they get there. So if at first you don't succeed – try again!

Accepting Anxiety

With this tip, we've come full circle, back to the top of the list: As we have stressed, having some anxiety is normal. It will keep returning. Welcome it with open arms. It means that you're still alive! Appreciate the positive aspects. Anxiety tells you to pay attention to what's going on around you. Go with the flow.

We're not suggesting that you need to feel overwhelming amounts of anxiety. But a little anxiety is unavoidable and may help you draw on your own resources during difficult challenges.

Chapter 22

Ten Signs That You Need Help – and Where to Get It

Some people find that self-help is all they need. They read about useful ways to deal with their anxiety, and then they apply what they've discovered. Lo and behold – their anxiety gradually fades to a manageable level.

However, no self-help book is intended to completely replace professional help. Anxiety sometimes requires the assistance of a professional, just as complicated tax matters may call for a qualified accountant, or to draw up your will you may want a solicitor. We hope you understand that seeking a mental health professional's assistance is a reasonable choice, not a sign of weakness.

This chapter tells you how to recognise if you should consider professional assistance for yourself or someone you care about. It's not always an obvious decision, so we give you a list of indicators. And if you still aren't sure, you can always talk with your GP, who should be able to help you decide.

We also tell you where you can find professional help, should you need it.

Having Suicidal Thoughts or Plans

You may be surprised to know that suicidal thoughts in themselves are not that uncommon. Recent research shows that up to 15 per cent of people in northern Europe may experience suicidal thoughts in any two-week period.

However, if you are having recurrent suicidal thoughts or have started to make plans to kill yourself, this needs to be taken very seriously and you should seek professional help straight away.

You can call the Samaritans on 08457 90 90 90 in the UK (local call rates) or, in the Republic of Ireland, dial 1850 60 90 90 (local call rates). Many Samaritans branches also offer local branch numbers. You can also use the Samaritans textphones (for the deaf and hard of hearing): Dial 08457 90 91 92 in the UK.

Alternatively, phone your GP – there are out-of-hours surgery numbers on the answerphone when the surgery is closed. NHS Direct is available by phone 24 hours a day; telephone 0845 4647. You can also call a friend.

If your thoughts become overwhelming, call 999 or go the accident and emergency (casualty) department at your nearest hospital. Help is available. There are people out there who care and know how to help you, and you don't have to be alone feeling this way. Don't be frightened to admit to people the truth about how you feel. It's nothing to be ashamed of, and with some support, you can feel better And when you do access professional help, be honest about your thoughts; hold nothing back.

Feeling Hopeless

From time to time, everyone feels defeated. But if you begin to feel hopeless about getting better, thinking that the future looks bleak and you can't do much to change it, get professional help. Feelings of hopelessness put you at greater risk of suicidal thoughts. But you need to know that you *can* feel better. Let others help you.

Feeling Both Anxious and Depressed

You may be experiencing depression mixed with anxiety if you find yourself having some of the following symptoms:

- Feeling sad most of the day
- Losing interest or pleasure in activities
- Loss of motivation
- Changes in weight
- Changes in your sleep patterns

✔ Feeling tense or, alternatively, lethargic

✔ Feeling worthless

✔ Feeling excessively guilty

✔ Poor concentration

✔ Thoughts of death

If you do have anxiety and depression, seek professional help. Depression is a treatable condition. Having the energy to fight both anxiety and depression at the same time can be pretty tough.

Trying – and Still Feeling Stuck

So you've read the book and given it your best shot to overcome anxiety, but for whatever reason, it just hasn't worked. That's okay. Don't get more anxious because you didn't get rid of worry and stress. Something else may be going on. Get an experienced mental health professional to help you figure out the next step.

Struggling at Home

You're anxious. The anxiety causes you to be irritable, jumpy, and upset. You just about cope at work and with strangers, but you take it out on the people you care about most, such as your family. Then you feel guilty, which increases your anxiety. If this sounds like you, a professional can help you decrease the tension at home and also find relief from your anxiety.

Dealing with Major Problems at Work

Maybe you have no-one at home to help you deal with your anxiety. Work stress can sometimes overwhelm you. If you find your anxiety exploding at work, consider professional help.

Anxiety can make you irritable and moody with colleagues or managers, and this can lead to problems. Anxiety can also affect your short-term memory and make it difficult to focus or to make decisions. So if anxiety impairs your ability to do your work, get help before things deteriorate.

Suffering from Severe Obsessions or Compulsions

Obsessive compulsive disorder (OCD) can be serious. See Chapter 2 for more information about OCD. The problem is that people with the disorder often don't seek help until their lives are ruled by unwanted thoughts or repetitive actions. Most people with OCD need professional help. If you or someone you love has more than mild OCD, get professional help.

Showing Signs of PTSD

You feel tense and agitated. Have you been caught up in a traumatic event?

- ✔ Did you feel helpless and afraid?
- ✔ Do you try not to think about it?
- ✔ In spite of your efforts not to think about it, do the thoughts and images keep on popping up?

If you've answered yes to these questions, you may have *post-traumatic stress disorder* (PTSD). See Chapter 2 for a complete description of PTSD. The treatment of PTSD is probably best left to an experienced professional. Many people with PTSD try to 'just get on with things' or 'keep a stiff upper lip' but find life is more limited because of their refusal to seek help. Don't let that be you.

Having Sleepless Nights

Is anxiety keeping you awake? That's quite common. If after working on your anxiety a while your sleep doesn't improve, be sure to read Chapter 11 about sleep. Too many sleepless nights make it hard to function and make it more difficult to help yourself in the fight against anxiety. If you sleep poorly night after night and wake tired, check it out with a professional. You may be experiencing depression along with anxiety.

Turning to Drink or Drugs

Excessive drinking or drug abuse can be a problem for those with anxiety disorders. It seems to makes sense, given that anxious feelings are uncomfortable.

But what begins as an innocent attempt to feel better can become a big problem later on. If you find yourself using too much alcohol or another drug to calm your feelings, get professional help before you become addicted.

Finding Help

To get professional help through the National Health Service (NHS), you usually go to your GP, who will be able to assess your difficulties and advise on treatment or referral to a psychiatrist or psychologist. You can normally request counselling, which is often available through your GP practice. It tends to be limited to around six sessions. Alternatively, there are some NHS centres where you can refer yourself, rather than only go to if your GP refers you.

Additional options include:

- ✔ Ask to be referred to a clinical psychologist or a psychiatrist. They normally work in community mental health teams (CMHTs). These teams often offer a range of psychological therapies, including cognitive behavioural therapy (CBT), the approach this book uses. Both the psychiatrist and your GP can prescribe medication.

- ✔ New developments in the NHS mean that stepped care is becoming available. Your GP can send you to the primary mental health team that is linked to your GP practice. From there, you may be referred on to the CMHT, which has closer links to a hospital.

- ✔ If you have private health insurance, this may include cover for psychological therapy. Once again, it is often best to go through your GP, but you will have a wider choice of specific therapists, and of therapies, including alternative or complementary ones such as homeopathy, acupuncture, reflexology, massage, and aromatherapy. You can also ask to see a medical herbalist.

- ✔ Insurance companies normally have a list of the practitioners they recognise. However, many therapists may not be on these lists, but still be appropriately qualified.

- ✔ Various professional organisations have lists of qualified practitioners. These organisations include the British Psychological Society, British Association of Behavioural and Cognitive Psychotherapy, and the United Kingdom Council for Psychotherapy (See the Appendix in the back of this book for more information).

We strongly recommend that you find out about the qualifications of anyone you would like to see, before making an appointment.

Appendix

Resources for You

• •

*I*n this Appendix, we provide some additional sources for finding out about and overcoming anxiety, as well as other emotional difficulties. These are only a few of the many excellent resources to supplement the information in this book.

Self-Help Books

Antony, Martin & Swinson, Richard. *The Shyness and Social Anxiety Workbook: Proven Techniques for Overcoming Your Fears.* Oakland: New Harbinger Publications, Inc., 2000.

Beckfield, Denise. *Master Your Panic and Take Back Your Life!* Atascadero: Impact Publishers, 2000.

Bien, Thomas & Bien, Beverly. *Mindful Recovery: A Spiritual Path to Healing from Addiction.* New York: John Wiley & Sons, Inc., 2002.

Bourne, Edmund. *The Anxiety and Phobia Workbook.* Oakland: New Harbinger Publications, Inc., 2000.

Burns, David. *The Feeling Good Handbook: Using the New Mood Therapy in Everyday Life.* New York: David Morrow and Company, Inc., 1989.

Carmin, Cheryl;*et al. Dying of Embarrassment: Help for Social Anxiety and Phobia.* Oakland: New Harbinger Publications, Inc., 1992.

Craske, Michelle; Barlow, David; & O'Leary, Tracy. *Mastery of Your Anxiety Land Worry.* San Antonio: The Psychological Corporation, 1992.

Davis, Martha; Eshelman, Elizabeth; & McKay, Matthew. *The Relaxation and Stress Reduction Workbook.* New York: MJF Books, 1995.

Elliott, Charles & Lassen, Maureen. *Why Can't I Get What I Want? How to Stop Making the Same Old Mistakes and Start Living a Life You Can Love.* Palo Alto: Davies-Black Publishing, 1998.

Ellis, Albert. *Feeling Better, Getting Better, Staying Better: Profound Self-Help Therapy for Your Emotions.* Atascadero: Impact Publishers, 2001.

Greenberger, Dennis & Padesky, Christine. *Mind Over Mood: Change How You Feel by Changing How You Think.* New York: The Guildford Press, 1995.

Jeffers, Susan. *Embracing Uncertainty.* London: Hodder & Stoughton, 2003.

Jeffers, Susan. *Feel the Fear and Do It Anyway.* London: Vermilion, imprint of Ebury Press, Random House, 2007.

Kabat-Zinn, Jon. *Full Catastrophe Living: Using the Wisdom of Your Body and Mind to Face Stress, Pain, and Illness.* New York: Bantam Doubleday Dell Publishing Group, Inc., 1990.

Luciani, Joseph. *Self-Coaching: How to Heal Anxiety and Depression.* New York: John Wiley & Sons, Inc., 2001.

Prochaska, James; Norcross, John; & DiClemente, Carlo. *Changing For Good: The Revolutionary Program that Explains the Six Stages of Change and Teaches you How to Free Yourself From Bad Habits.* New York: William Morrow & Co., Inc., 1994.

Ruiz, Don Miguel. *The Four Agreements.* California: Amber Allen Publishing Inc., 1997.

Servan-Schreiber, David. *Healing Without Freud or Prozac: Natural Approaches to Curing Stress, Anxiety and Depression.* London: Rodale International Limited, 2005.

Tolle, Eckhart. *The Power of Now.* London: Hodder & Stoughton, 2003.

Walker, Eugene. *Learn to Relax: Proven Techniques for Reducing Stress, Tension, and Anxiety – and Promoting Peak Performance.* New York: John Wiley & Sons, Inc., 2000.

Resources to Help Children

Chansky, Tamar. *Freeing Your Child From Obsessive-Compulsive Disorder: A Powerful, Practical Program for Parents of Children and Adolescents.* New York: Three Rivers Press, The Crown Publishing Group, 2001.

Clark, Lynn. *SOS Help for Parents.* Bowling Green: Parents' Press, 1996.

Elliott, Charles & Smith, Laura. *Why Can't I Be the Parent I Want to Be? End Old Patterns and Enjoy Your Children.* Oakland: New Harbinger Publications, Inc., 1999.

Manassis, Katharina. *Keys to Parenting Your Anxious Child.* Hauppauge: Barrans Educational Series, 1996.

Rapee, Ronald (Ed.) *et al.Helping Your Anxious Child: A Step-By-Step Guide for Parents.* Oakland: New Harbinger Publications, Inc., 2000.

Schaefer, Charles. *Cats Got Your Tongue? A Story for Children Afraid to Speak.* Washington, D.C.: Magination, American Psychological Association, 1992.

Smith, Laura & Elliott, Charles. *Hollow Kids: Recapturing the Soul of a Generation Lost to the Self-Esteem Myth.* Roseville: Prima Publishing Division of Random House, 2001.

Accessing Web Sites to Discover More about Anxiety

Type the word *anxiety* into a search engine, and literally thousands of sites pop up. Be careful. The Web is contains both unscrupulous sales pitches and misinformation, and also extremely valuable, accurate information. Be especially cautious about official-sounding organisations that promote materials for sale. Don't be fooled by instant cures for anxiety.

Many Web forums host chat rooms for people suffering from anxiety. Be careful about accessing them for support, as you don't know anything for certain about who these people really are, and some may try to take advantage of your distress. Don't believe everything you read.

There are plenty of Web sites around the world you can access on the Internet. Here's a list of a variety of legitimate Web sites based in the UK:

- ✔ **The National Phobics Society** (www.phobics-society.org.uk) is the largest UK charity for people affected by anxiety disorders. It is a user-led organisation that works to relieve and support those living with anxiety disorders by providing information, support, and understanding via an extensive range of services, including one-to-one therapy services. It also works regularly with external agencies and healthcare professionals to improve the service provision offered to those living with anxiety disorders, and campaigns to raise awareness of anxiety disorders through holding events like the annual Anxiety Disorders Awareness Week. The organisation also has a helpline: 0870 122 2325 – Monday to Friday 9.15 a.m. – 9 p.m.

- ✔ **No More Panic** (www.nomorepanic.co.uk) provides valuable information for sufferers and carers of people with panic, anxiety, phobias and Obsessive Compulsive Disorder (OCD).

- ✔ **The National Institute for Mental Health In England** (www.patient.co.uk) reports on research about a wide variety of mental health issues. They also have an array of educational materials on anxiety. They provide resources for researchers and practitioners in the field.

- ✔ **The British Psychological Society** (www.bps.org.uk) provides a list of qualified psychologists, and areas of specialty.

- ✔ **The British Association of Behavioural and Cognitive Psychotherapies** (www.babcp.com) has information for the public about anxiety and other mental disorders, and has a list of qualified psychotherapists with their areas of expertise.

Index

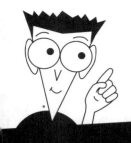

FOR DUMMIES

Do Anything. Just Add Dummies

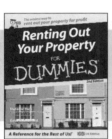 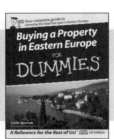 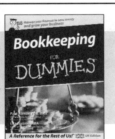

Buying and Selling a Home FOR DUMMIES
978-0-7645-7027-8

Renting Out Your Property FOR DUMMIES
978-0-470-02921-3

Buying a Property in Eastern Europe FOR DUMMIES
978-0-7645-7047-6

RSONAL FINANCE

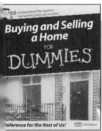 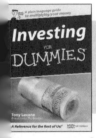 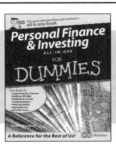

Investing FOR DUMMIES
978-0-7645-7023-0

Personal Finance & Investing ALL-IN-ONE FOR DUMMIES
978-0-470-51510-5

Bookkeeping FOR DUMMIES
978-0-470-05815-2

INESS

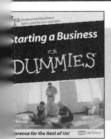 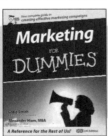 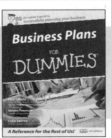

Starting a Business FOR DUMMIES
978-0-7645-7018-6

Marketing FOR DUMMIES
978-0-7645-7056-8

Business Plans FOR DUMMIES
978-0-7645-7026-1

Answering Tough Interview Questions For Dummies (978-0-470-01903-0)

Arthritis For Dummies (978-0-470-02582-6)

Being the Best Man For Dummies (978-0-470-02657-1)

British History For Dummies (978-0-470-03536-8)

Building Self-Confidence For Dummies (978-0-470-01669-5)

Buying a Home on a Budget For Dummies (978-0-7645-7035-3)

Children's Health For Dummies (978-0-470-02735-6)

Cognitive Behavioural Therapy For Dummies (978-0-470-01838-5)

Cricket For Dummies (978-0-470-03454-5)

CVs For Dummies (978-0-7645-7017-9)

Detox For Dummies (978-0-470-01908-5)

Diabetes For Dummies (978-0-470-05810-7)

Divorce For Dummies (978-0-7645-7030-8)

DJing For Dummies (978-0-470-03275-6)

eBay.co.uk For Dummies (978-0-7645-7059-9)

English Grammar For Dummies (978-0-470-05752-0)

Gardening For Dummies (978-0-470-01843-9)

Genealogy Online For Dummies (978-0-7645-7061-2)

Green Living For Dummies (978-0-470-06038-4)

Hypnotherapy For Dummies (978-0-470-01930-6)

Life Coaching For Dummies (978-0-470-03135-3)

Neuro-linguistic Programming For Dummies (978-0-7645-7028-5)

Nutrition For Dummies (978-0-7645-7058-2)

Parenting For Dummies (978-0-470-02714-1)

Pregnancy For Dummies (978-0-7645-7042-1)

Rugby Union For Dummies (978-0-470-03537-5)

Self Build and Renovation For Dummies (978-0-470-02586-4)

Starting a Business on eBay.co.uk For Dummies (978-0-470-02666-3)

Starting and Running an Online Business For Dummies (978-0-470-05768-1)

The GL Diet For Dummies (978-0-470-02753-0)

The Romans For Dummies (978-0-470-03077-6)

Thyroid For Dummies (978-0-470-03172-8)

UK Law and Your Rights For Dummies (978-0-470-02796-7)

Writing a Novel and Getting Published For Dummies (978-0-470-05910-4)

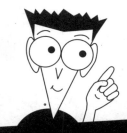

FOR DUMMIES®

Do Anything. Just Add Dummies

HOBBIES

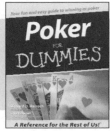

978-0-7645-5232-8

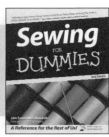

978-0-7645-6847-3

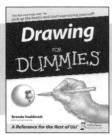

978-0-7645-5476-6

Also available:

Art For Dummies
(978-0-7645-5104-8)
Aromatherapy For Dummies
(978-0-7645-5171-0)
Bridge For Dummies
(978-0-471-92426-5)
Card Games For Dummies
(978-0-7645-9910-1)
Chess For Dummies
(978-0-7645-8404-6)

Improving Your Memory
For Dummies
(978-0-7645-5435-3)
Massage For Dummies
(978-0-7645-5172-7)
Meditation For Dummies
(978-0-471-77774-8)
Photography For Dummi
(978-0-7645-4116-2)
Quilting For Dummies
(978-0-7645-9799-2)

EDUCATION

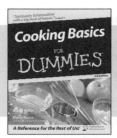

978-0-7645-7206-7

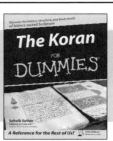

978-0-7645-5581-7

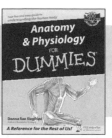

978-0-7645-5422-3

Also available:

Algebra For Dummies
(978-0-7645-5325-7)
Algebra II For Dummies
(978-0-471-77581-2)
Astronomy For Dummies
(978-0-7645-8465-7)
Buddhism For Dummies
(978-0-7645-5359-2)
Calculus For Dummies
(978-0-7645-2498-1)

Forensics For Dummies
(978-0-7645-5580-0)
Islam For Dummies
(978-0-7645-5503-9)
Philosophy For Dummie
(978-0-7645-5153-6)
Religion For Dummies
(978-0-7645-5264-9)
Trigonometry For Dumr
(978-0-7645-6903-6)

PETS

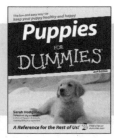

978-0-470-03717-1

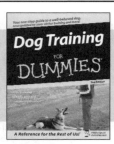

978-0-7645-8418-3

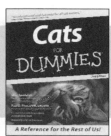

978-0-7645-5275-5

Also available:

Labrador Retrievers
For Dummies
(978-0-7645-5281-6)
Aquariums For Dummies
(978-0-7645-5156-7)
Birds For Dummies
(978-0-7645-5139-0)
Dogs For Dummies
(978-0-7645-5274-8)
Ferrets For Dummies
(978-0-7645-5259-5)

Golden Retrievers
For Dummies
(978-0-7645-5267-0)
Horses For Dummies
(978-0-7645-9797-8)
Jack Russell Terriers
For Dummies
(978-0-7645-5268-7)
Puppies Raising & Train
Diary For Dummies
(978-0-7645-0876-9)